Compacts and Cosmetics:

Beauty from Victorian Times to the Present Day

Dedication

For John and Josh who live with my collecting passion and my mother, Nicolette Marsh, who inspired it.

Compacts and Cosmetics:

Beauty from Victorian Times to the Present Day

By Madeleine Marsh

Women with Style Series

Acknowledgements

Collecting and learning about objects is a collaborative process. I would like to thank the many women (and some men) who shared their make-up memories with me. I am grateful to family and friends who ransacked drawers and bathroom cupboards to contribute to my collection. Thanks are due to the staff at Chelsea Library (a user-friendly treasure trove of fashion journals) and to the dealers who gave me generous help and advice, in particular Linda Bee and Gray's Antiques Market in London. Invaluable assistance was also provided by Matthew Blurton, Roger Hyams and John Arcedeckne Butler.

Lipstick kisses to all concerned.

First published in Great Britain in 2009 by
REMEMBER WHEN
An imprint of
Pen & Sword Books Ltd
47 Church Street
Barnsley
South Yorkshire
S70 2AS

Copyright © Madeleine Marsh 2009

ISBN 978 18446 804 98

Typeset by Mac Style, Beverley, East Yorkshire
Printed and bound by 1010 Printing International Ltd.

Pen & Sword Books Ltd incorporates the Imprints of Pen & Sword Aviation, Pen & Sword Maritime, Pen & Sword Military, Wharncliffe Local History, Pen & Sword Select, Pen & Sword Military Classics, Leo Cooper, Remember When, Seaforth Publishing and Frontline Publishing.

For a complete list of Pen & Sword titles please contact
PEN & SWORD BOOKS LIMITED
47 Church Street, Barnsley, South Yorkshire, S70 2AS, England
E-mail: enquiries@pen-and-sword.co.uk
Website: www.pen-and-sword.co.uk

Contents

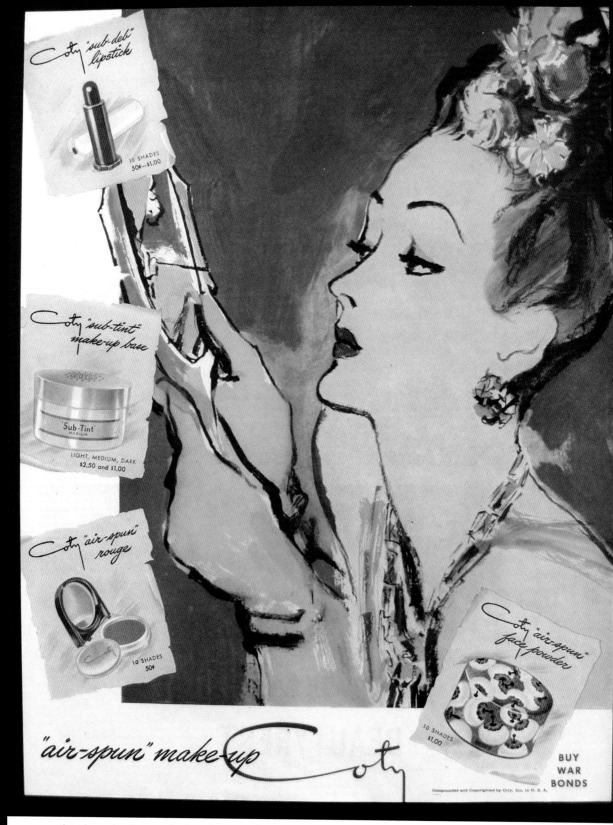

American advertisement for Coty air-spun make-up with added instruction to 'Buy War Bonds' dating from the Second World War.

Introduction

'I'VE GOT TO put a face on,' my mother would always say before preparing to go out for the evening. As a child, this expression confused me. Surely she had a face already? Who was forcing her to put on another one? And how different she looked, felt and smelt when she kissed me goodnight in her sticky pink lipstick, feathery false eyelashes and the scratchy silver face-glitter that matched her silver wig and lurex maxi dress. This was, after all, the late 1960s and we lived in swinging London.

As an adult, the phrase still fascinates me. Putting a face on marks the division between one's private and public self; between what we look like naturally and how we wish to appear to the world: smoother, younger, bigger-eyed, brighter-lipped, more professional, more fashionable, more desirable …

It also – generally speaking – marks the division between men and women. Though at the time of writing the male grooming market is booming and the chemist chain Superdrug has just launched a new beauty range for metrosexual man including 'Manscara' and 'Guyliner'; most typically cosmetics are reserved for women. Like high heels and body-shaping underwear, make-up is part of a semi-secret armoury that helps us change our appearance and emphasise our femininity. And like these constricting fashion accessories (great to put on and a relief to take off) it is both a blessing and a curse.

One of the joys of being female is the freedom to transform your look. For little girls experimenting with lipstick and eyeshadow is part of the initiation ceremony into a grown-up world of bras and boyfriends and whatever your age, playing with make-up is fun. You can be decorative and creative; you can ally yourself with different tribes from Goths to immaculately groomed celebrities. Most importantly – you can emphasise your best bits and conceal the worst ones and that is where the paradox begins.

Even as a child I somehow understood that my mother's phrase implied a sense of obligation. Whatever women do at home, they are often expected (and expect themselves) to put on a face in public. On the one hand make-up is empowering – the better you look, the better you feel and the better you do. 'Put your best face forward,' advised cosmetics advertisements during World War II. 'Look your Best to Do your Best.'

On the other hand, this also implies that without a concealing film of tinted fats and powders (to say nothing of depilation, moisturising, deodorising and all the other traditional, tedious and occasionally dangerous feminine beauty practises) you are less attractive, less capable, less worthy, and ultimately less of a woman. Across the Twentieth Century cosmetics were increasingly portrayed not just as a pleasure but a duty. Edwardian beauty guides instructed ladies to avoid 'the sin of dowdiness'; 1930s magazines warned wives that if they 'let themselves go', then their husbands would leave too. By the 1970s, feminists were instructing sisters to throw away cosmetics (along with bras, depilatories and husbands) and having cast off the patriarchal chains of artificial beauty to rejoice in their natural, unpainted hairy selves. Fat chance …

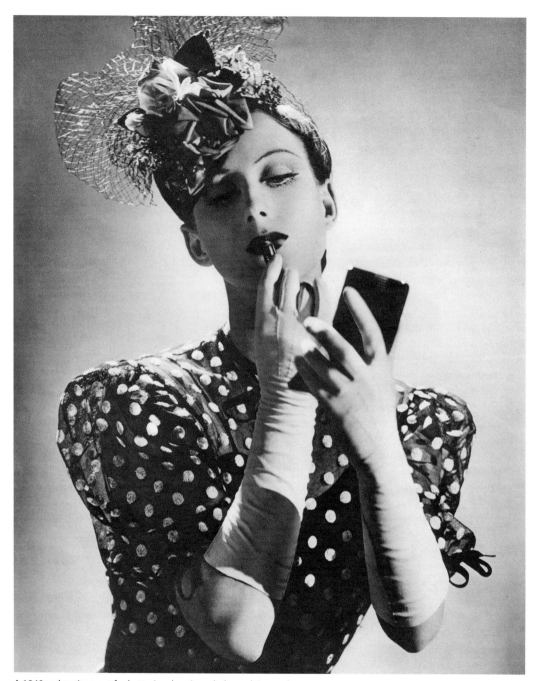

A 1940s advertisement for batteries showing a lady applying make-up.

Thirty years on a paparazzi shot of a Hollywood star revealing a fuzzy armpit or a tired, make-up free face, is still regarded as shocking enough to appear in gossip magazines across the world. In Britain alone, consumers spend over £16 billion a year on health and beauty products; and though they might be sexually liberated and financially independent, nothing it seems can separate women from their make-up bags.

Though it might not be a physical necessity, make-up is certainly a psychological essential. In the course of writing this book I talked to several women who would have felt more comfortable going out without knickers than lipstick. 'I wear it all the time, even when I'm on my own at home,' explained one. 'I feel naked without my bright red lips.' Another recurring topic was when you could first allow a partner to see you without make-up. For some sleeping with a new man was somehow easier and less intimate than appearing bare faced the morning after, and many admitted to creeping out of bed first thing to secretly reapply last night's party face.

The word make-up originated in the theatre and the overtones of make-believe and deception – putting a face on to pretend to be someone you're not – go someway to explaining why across the centuries men have had an ambivalent attitude towards cosmetics. Like animals in the mating season women colour their skin in part to attract the male, but woe betide them if they are unmasked. In his 1732 poem *The Lady's Dressing Room*, Jonathan Swift mocked the despair of the romantic Strephon, who searching the chambers of the beauteous Celia (a woman who takes an impressive five hours getting ready), uncovers a plethora of 'ointments, daubs, paints and creams'; a pair of tweezers for dealing with those embarrassing stray hairs; her smelly stockings and soiled underwear. Horrified by Celia's concealing cosmetics and her oozing, reeking humanity Strephon is put off women for life.

Too much 'slap' (another theatrical term, deriving from slapping on the greasepaint) and a girl can be condemned as a slapper. In the Eighteenth Century – when women blanched their complexions with white lead and hid pockmarks under decorative patches – men's fear of deception reached its zenith, so much so that in 1770 Parliament passed an act decreeing that any woman who sought to betray one of His Majesty's subjects into marriage by 'scents, paints, cosmetic washes, artificial teeth, false hair, Spanish wool (rouge), iron stays, high-heeled shoes, bolstered hips and like misdemeanours shall incur the penalty of the law in force against witchcraft and that marriage shall stand null and void.'

Reacting against the excesses of the Eighteenth Century – and the threat of lead poisoning and divorce – the Victorian lady was expected to be entirely cosmetic free, her unpainted face reflecting her inner virtue. But you can't keep a good woman down (let alone a bad one).

This book explores the history of make-up and beauty in western culture from the Nineteenth Century to the modern age: what we did to our faces and bodies, why we did it and who we wanted to look like.

Beginning in the Victorian age, when 'painted lady' was a euphemism for prostitute and a respectable girl was supposed to restrict herself to a dab of cold cream, it explores the origins of the mass-produced beauty business (soaps, creams, hair care, etc.), and the birth of some of today's most famous brand names.

Moving into the 1900s it chronicles the rise of the modern cosmetics industry and tells the story of some of the great pioneers; Elizabeth Arden, Max Factor, Helena Rubinstein, who helped transform make-up from a guilty secret into an every day handbag essential, and literally changed the face of the century.

Across the Twentieth Century, this chronological survey shows how make-up expresses the needs of the times – both in peace and war – and how what we do to our faces and bodies reflects the fashions of the day and the changing roles of men and women. It identifies period icons from flappers to film stars to supermodels, and charts cosmetic innovations from the twist-up lipstick to the aerosol hairspray.

Each chapter uncovers the secret life and personal grooming habits of women over the decades and is illustrated with favourite dressing table accessories of the day from glamorous powder compacts to discreet lady shaves. Vintage beauty items and ephemera are now popular collectables and this book also provides a collector's guide to compacts and cosmetic accessories – revealing the make-up that you shouldn't throw away once it's past its sell-by date.

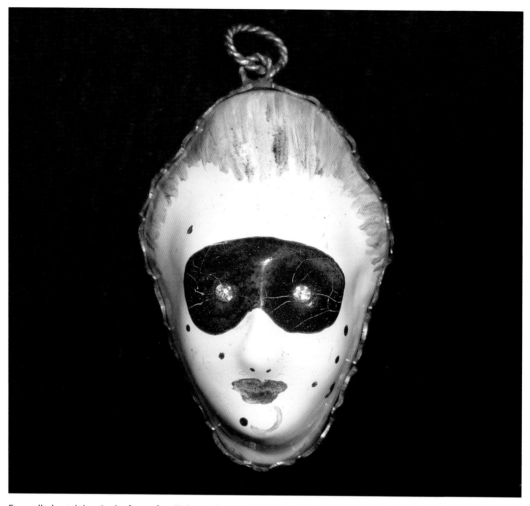

Enamelled patch box in the form of an Eighteenth Century lady with white lead painted face and patches.

The final chapter focuses on the present when with fears about the lasting effects of botox and cosmetic surgery, the rise of tattooing and piercing, and the demands posed by an ageing population, what we do to our bodies remains a controversial topic.

In theory at least we've travelled a long way from the Victorian dressing table and at the dawn of the new millennium, we have more products to choose from than ever before. (Do you know how much make-up you own? Would you be surprised by the number of items and horrified if you totted up the total cost?)

Mass-produced cosmetics and the luxury of choice might be a comparatively modern phenomenon but the urge to decorate the skin is as old as time itself and the introductory chapter goes back to the ancient world to explore the first recorded use of cosmetics and the literal foundation of make-up.

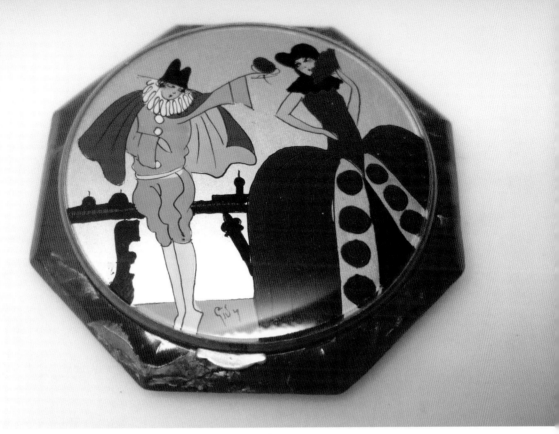

1920s handpainted compact, made in France. *Gray's Antiques Market*

A collection of modern make-up and beauty products – fifteen items used to put on a Twenty-first Century face.

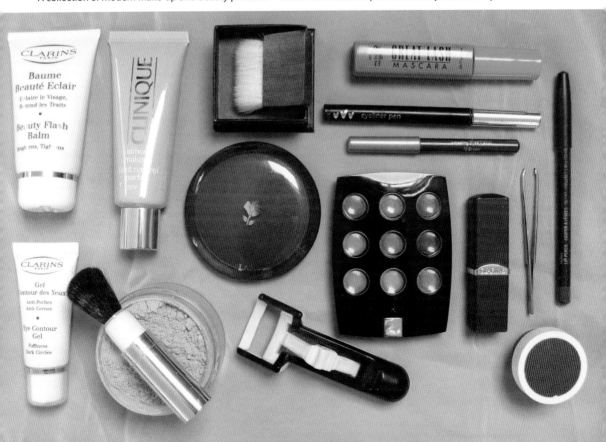

CHAPTER ONE

The Foundation of Make-up

Beauty in the Ancient World

F ROM THE DAWN of time men and women have decorated their bodies. Prehistoric peoples painted and scarified the skin to indicate tribal allegiance, to scare their enemies, and honour their gods but the first recorded use of make-up for pleasure derives from Ancient Egypt.

Egypt

The Egyptians pioneered the development of cosmetics and fragrances. They lived and died surrounded by kohl jars, make-up boxes, perfume vials and polished metal mirrors, all of which were buried with them to provide eternal beauty in the afterlife. They painted their eyes, rouged their lips, spent hours arranging their hairstyles, and many of the time-consuming grooming practises that we take for granted today were established four thousand years ago on the banks of the Nile.

Depilation and Moisturising

A smooth skin was highly prized and body hair was removed with pumice stones, tweezers, and bronze razors, all of which have been found in tombs. The Hearst Medical Papyrus (a list of cures and remedies inscribed in the second millennium BC) recommended a concoction of heated lard, insect droppings and boiled bird bones as a wax depilatory, or more simply suggested rubbing the offending hair with blood from the vulva of a female greyhound.

In a harsh, hot climate moisturising the body was practised by every class. When Howard Carter opened up Tutankhamen's tomb in 1922, he discovered sealed jars containing traces of scented skin cream that was still fragrant after 3,000 years. At the other end of the social scale, during the reign of Rameses III when the tomb builders of Deir el-Medina laid down tools (one of history's first recorded strikes), a major cause of their pioneering industrial action was the non-supply of castor and sesame oils, which were an agreed part of their monthly rations and essential for keeping the skin supple in desert conditions.

Eye paint and Face make-up

Make-up was used both for prophylactic and decorative purposes. Thick lines of eye paint helped protect the eyes from the sun's glare and powdered kohl was also included in eye medicines. Worn by both men and women, eye paint came in two main colours – green made from malachite (copper carbonate) and black from galena (lead sulphide). Ingredients were ground on a cosmetic palette, mixed with oil or water, then applied to the eyes either with the fingers or a kohl pencil – a slim stick sometimes with a small mixing spoon or spatula at one end. Kohl pots came in a range of styles from small alabaster boxes to long slender glass tubes, and containers were often decorated with the image of Bes – protector of the household, pregnant women and children, and the deity associated with pleasure. Decorating the eyes also had a symbolic value, simulating the eye of Horus (the falcon god) and providing a protective amulet against the evil eye.

Yellow ochre paint was used to lighten the skin (men also used a darker orange tone); red ochre was powdered to rouge the lips and cheeks. The Turin Erotic Papyrus – the Ancient Egyptian equivalent of a girlie magazine and a monument to human athleticism and sexual invention during the Rameses' period (1292-1075BC) – includes the illustration of a female nude, straddling a vast phallus whilst calmly painting her mouth; lip brush in one hand, mirror and cosmetic tube in the other. Like Twentieth Century pin-ups, even if you had no clothes on, you needed to be sure that your make-up was flawless.

Skin Decoration and Tattooing
Henna was used to tint fingernails and decorate the skin; more permanent markings were provided by puncture tattooing. According to evidence from mummies and statuettes, tattooing appears to have been largely restricted to women including dancers and concubines. Geometric designs were inked on the body (often around the stomach area) whilst the inner thigh was tattooed with representations of Bes, a good luck charm whether you wanted to ward off sexual disease or ensure a safe labour.

Hair care
Henna also served to colour the hair and medical papyri included numerous recipes for hair dyes and scalp treatments. Donkey liver, or a cooked mouse – left to rot then mixed with lard – provided a salve that would prevent greyness. Another remedy suggested strengthening the hair with the juice of a black lizard boiled in oil, whilst baldness could be cured with a pomade of fat extracted from the lion, the hippo, the crocodile, the tomcat, the snake and the Nubian ibex.

Small wonder perhaps that shaving the head was a popular alternative. 'The priests shave themselves all over their body every other day, so that no lice or any other foul thing may come to be upon them when they minister to the gods,' observed the Fifth Century BC Greek historian Herodotus.

At various periods civilian men, and women too, shaved their heads, resorting to elaborate wigs that could be styled and beeswaxed into the latest fashionable shapes. Another artificial favourite was a long and slender false beard worn by both male and female pharaohs as a symbol of status. Tomb paintings show ladies supporting cones of fat upon their heads, which according to one explanation were designed to melt as the evening progressed, thus moisturising their wigs. A less messy theory was that these cones were a hieroglyphic symbol, indicating that their hairpieces were richly perfumed.

Perfume
Fragrance was used for both cosmetic and religious purposes. The word perfume comes from the Latin *per fumum*: through smoke. Across the Ancient World incense was burnt in temples to appease the gods, to raise the soul to the heavens and to conceal the all too earthy smells of sacrificed flesh and an unwashed congregation. Perfume was inseparable from love, life and death. As Shakespeare tells it Cleopatra seduced Mark Antony on a barge with scented purple sails 'so perfumèd that the winds were love-sick with them'. Corpses were embalmed with myrrh and cassia and wrapped in scented bandages both as a symbol of eternity and to preserve the body from putrefaction.

Ancient Greece

Perfume and cosmetics (often imported from Egypt and the Far East) spread across the Mediterranean. In Athens, women rouged their cheeks with cinnabar (red mercury sulphide) and blanched their complexions with powdered white lead, products which as the Roman naturalist Pliny observed were 'deadly poisons'. Despite persistent warnings, lead continued to be used in cosmetics until well into the Nineteenth Century and from deadly nightshade – used in ancient times to dilate the pupils (hence its Italian name belladonna: beautiful lady) – to modern day botox (smoothing out wrinkles with *botulinus toxin*), poisonous substances have remained a constituent of make-up.

It wasn't just women who were dying to be beautiful. In Athens, a culture that venerated the male body, moisturising the skin was an important part of the masculine bathing process, as described by the poet Antiphanes in the Fourth Century BC.

'He really bathes
In a large gilded tub, and steeps his feet
And legs in rich Egyptian unguents;
His neck and chest he rubs with oil of palm
And both his arms with extract of sweet mint,
His eyebrows and his hair with Marjoram,
His knees and face with essence of ground thyme.'

Socrates rejected such perfumed foppery declaring that the only scent a man needed was 'nobility of soul' and in warlike Sparta cosmetics and fragrances were banned.

Rome

Warlike Rome however embraced them with enthusiasm. In his *Natural History* (77AD), Pliny noted with disgust that soldiers had taken to wearing perfume underneath their helmets and that even the standards and eagles of the Legions, the emblems of Roman power across the world, were steeped in scented oils, providing a fragrant symbol of 'our state of extreme corruptness'.

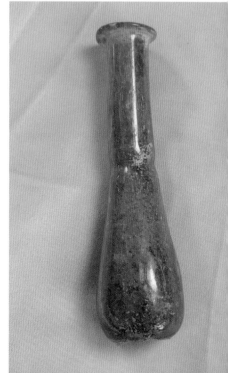

Pliny criticised the vast amounts of money wasted on cosmetic unguents, the most fugitive and as such 'the most superfluous' of luxuries. Nero was famous for his love of expensive fragrances, even perfuming (reports Pliny despairingly) the soles of his feet. Silver pipes were installed in the imperial palace to spray visitors with rosewater and on one occasion the emperor spent a fortune on a waterfall of rose petals, that smothered and killed one of his guests. Nero's wife (and former mistress) Poppaea Sabina was said to bathe daily in milk from her personal herd of 500 asses, and devised her own pomatums to guard against wrinkles.

Roman matrons covered themselves in make-up. In Book III of *Ars Amatoria* (The Art of Love) the Roman poet Ovid offered frank advice to women on every subject from how to fake an orgasm ('don't betray yourself by over-acting') to personal grooming.

Roman glass bottle for oil and cosmetics dating from the First or Second Century, AD.

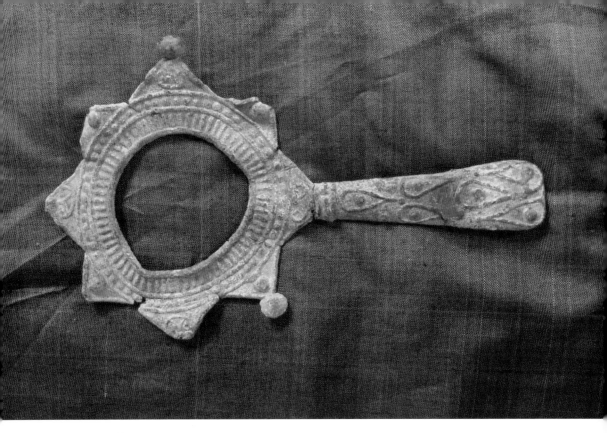

Roman lead frame for a hand mirror.

West African bronze kohl stick and tazolt kohl stone. Tazolt is a stone found in Taoudeni (700 Kms North of Timbuktu). When scratched with a stick, or ground to a powder it creates natural kohl or eye make-up. The Tuareg people have used tazolt for centuries and well as being worn by women it is traditionally used by 'Marabouts' (Islamic leaders and scholars) to protect their eyes from the sun whilst studying religious texts.

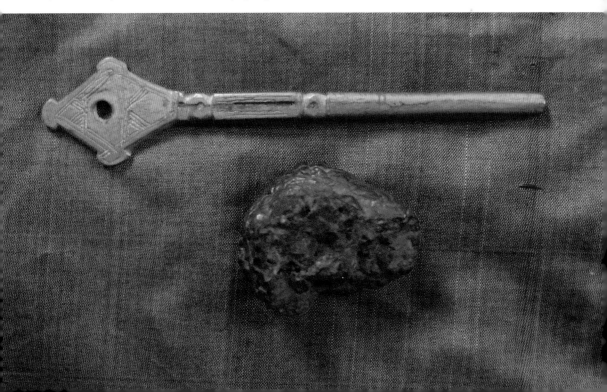

Stinking armpits and bristly legs were, he emphasised, to be avoided at all cost. Chalk was recommended for whitening the skin, carmine for pinking the cheeks and powdered ash and saffron for emphasising the eyes. If you were not fortunate enough to have a mono-brow (much prized in Ancient Rome and Greece) Ovid suggests inking one in; similarly thin hair could be rectified by wigs; and patches could be used to conceal spots and blemishes. As far as Ovid was concerned there was nothing at all wrong with make-up and artificial embellishments, so long as they were applied in secret:

> 'On no account let your lover find you with a lot of "aids to beauty" boxes about you. The art that adorns you should be unsuspected … Let your servants tell us you are still asleep, if we arrive before your toilet is finished. You will appear all the lovelier when you've put on the finishing touch. Why should I know what it is that makes your skin so white? Keep your door shut, and don't let me see the work before it's finished. There are a whole host of things we men should know nothing about.'

Whereas in Ancient Egypt men and women alike showed off their cosmetic accessories and revelled in obviously artificial make-up and false hair; the beauties of Rome were expected to 'appear' natural and were mocked if they were caught out.

'You dye you hair, but never will you dye your old age … Never will rouge or white paint turn Hecuba into Helen,' warned the Second Century Greek writer Lucian. 'Your hair was made far away and at night you put away your teeth in the same manner as your silks. You lie stored away in a hundred little cosmetic boxes – your face doesn't even sleep with you,' sneered the poet Martial in his epigrams. Even the liberal Ovid had no patience with men who experimented with make-up. 'Don't, for heaven's sake, have your hair waved, or use powder on your skin,' urged the so-called 'Master of Love' who recommended that gentlemen should confine themselves to a decent hair cut and a good wash ('don't go about reeking like a billy goat'). Men should, he adds, remember to clean their teeth, manicure their nails and trim their nose hair but 'All other toilet refinements leave to the women or to perverts.'

Ungodly make-up

It wasn't just Roman satirists who attacked the wearing of obvious make-up. With the rise of Christianity and the collapse of unguent-guzzling Rome, cosmetics and perfumes were stigmatised as sinful luxuries. In the bible Jezebel, the pagan queen of Israel, was demonised not just for cruelly subjugating the Jews, but for painting her face and fixing her hair; her name becoming a synonym for prostitute across the millennia. Saints and early Christian converts condemned any attempt whatsoever to improve upon God's creation. 'What place has rouge and white lead on the face of a Christian woman?' demanded St Jerome in his letters. '… They serve only to inflame young men's passions, to stimulate lust and to indicate an unchaste mind.' 'Women in general should be warned that the work of God … should in no way be falsified by employing yellow colouring or black powder or rouge, or, finally, any cosmetic at all that spoils the natural features,' insisted St Cyprian. 'Everything that comes into existence is the work of God; whatever is changed, is the work of the devil.'

By the start of the first millennium, the basic paradox of make-up was already established. From Ancient Egypt came a wealth of cosmetics and grooming practices, many of which are still the accepted norm today. The Romans encouraged women to apply their make-up in secret and to use it to simulate natural perfection. The early Christians ordered them to reject cosmetics altogether, dismissing them as deceitful, immoral and a source of shame.

The following history of cosmetics and beauty begins nearly 2,000 years on in the Nineteenth Century, but for the Victorian ladies sitting at their dressing tables, the conflict between natural and artificial beauty was not only still raging, it was at its height.

Chapter Two

Unpainted Ladies

Beauty in the Victorian Age

FOR THE VICTORIAN lady – thanks to the industrial revolution and heightened moral sensibility – fashion became a virtual prison. The period ideal of fragile, fainting femininity was rendered almost inevitable by new developments in underwear. With the invention of metal eyelets in the 1820s stays could be laced tighter than ever before, squeezing the waist with steel and whalebone. The corset is 'a tyrant – that aspiring to embrace, hugs like a bear – crushing in the ribs, injuring the lungs and heart, the stomach and many other internal organs,' fumed Mary Eliza Haweis in *The Art of Beauty 1878*. 'And all to what end? The end of looking like a wasp, and losing the whole charm of graceful human movement and easy carriage – the end of communicating an over-all-ish sense of deformity!'

A tiny waist was set off by an enormous skirt, initially supported by heavy layers of petticoats, then from the 1850s by the crinoline – a literal cage of steel hoops that could give a woman a six-foot circumference. The metal crinoline might have been lighter and cooler than scratchy linen and horsehair underskirts, but it was scarcely more liberating. 'Kind feeling alone ought to put an end to this stupid fashion which makes our dress a nuisance in every railway carriage, omnibus and pew, and all other places where the sitting room is small,' grumbled the *Alexandra Magazine* in 1864.

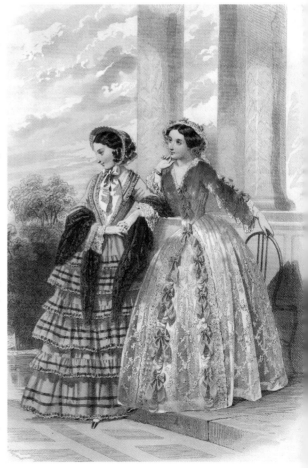

Les Modes Parisiennes – French fashion print, 1852.

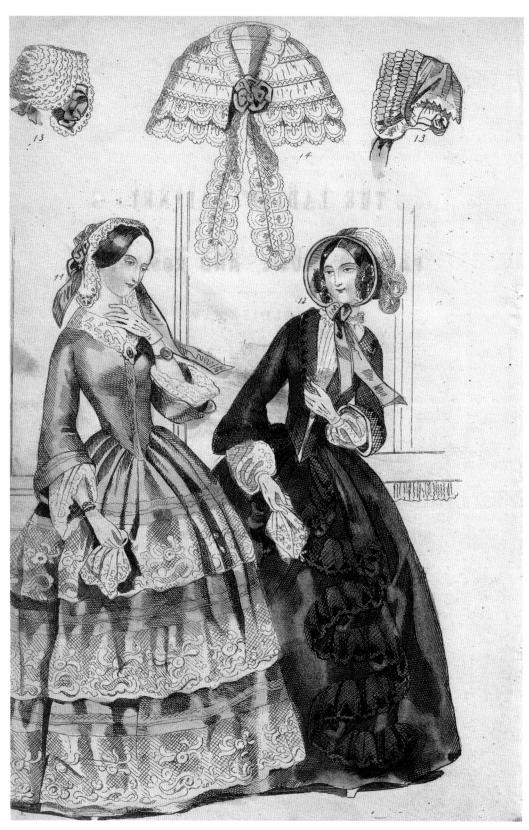

Victorian fashion print, 1850s.

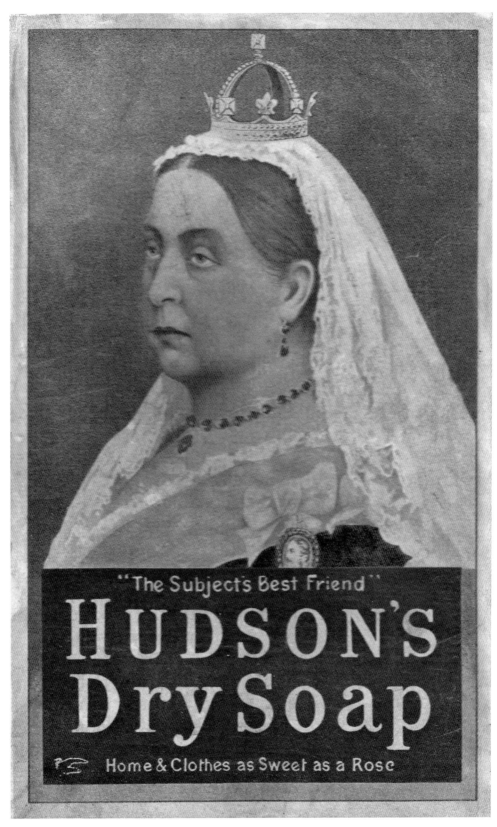

Victorian advertising showcard for Hudson's Dry Soap.

It was also potentially dangerous. Newspapers reported horror stories about girls getting trapped in machinery and the fireplace was a constant hazard. 'We never see a lady on the hearthrug, without fearing she will make an *auto da fe* of herself,' mocked *Punch* magazine in 1859. 'We have put down in India the practice of *Suttee*, but in England wives and daughters are consumed as well as widows … Lives enough are lost through their shoes and tight-lacing, without our adding Crinoline as a depopulating influence.'

From her toes scrunched up in pointy buttoned boots to the tips of her fingers squeezed in tight kid gloves the Victorian lady was expected to sacrifice comfort for constraint. The fashionable silhouette was immobilising and rampantly artificial, but the one area of the body where, in theory at least, no artifice was allowed was the face.

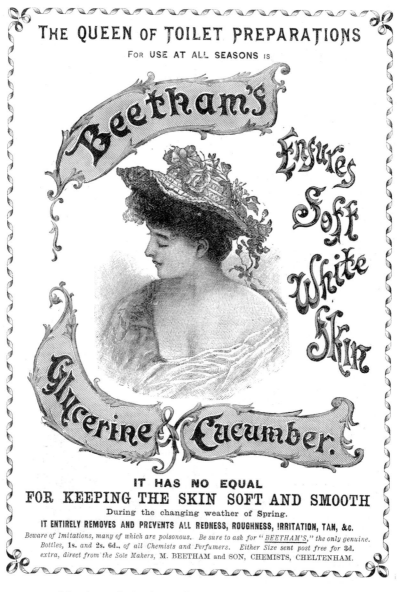

Advertisment for Beetham's Glycerine & Cucumber Lotion, c.1900.

Unpainted ladies

Obvious use of make-up was considered indecent and face painting was dismissed as the preserve of actresses and streetwalkers (hence the expression painted lady). 'If Satan has ever had any direct agency in inducing woman to spoil or deform her own beauty, it must have been in tempting her to use paints and enamelling. Ladies ought to know that it is a sure spoiler of the skin, and good taste ought to teach them that it is a frightful distorter and deformer of the natural beauty of the 'human face divine', warned Lola Montez in 1858, who as an exotic dancer and famous courtesan herself might be expected to know a thing or two about the evils of cosmetics.

The classic image of Victorian beauty – a peaches and cream complexion, cherry ripe lips, a pair of sparkling eyes fringed by soft, fluttering lashes – was expected to be natural, a gift from God. Despite any evidence to the contrary, external loveliness was associated with inner virtue. Fashion guides stressed the cosmetic benefits of early rising, cold water, fresh air and temperance. According to the most extreme opponents of cosmetics 'plain living and high thinking' would do more for the skin than powder and paint, and improving the mind was a sure-fire way of improving the appearance.

Lola, writing in the intriguingly titled *The Arts of Beauty: or, Secrets of a Lady's Toilet With Hints to Gentlemen on the Art of Fascinating* was a little more circumspect: 'It is true that a beautiful mind is the first thing requisite for a beautiful face, yet how much more charming will the whole become through the aid of a fine complexion!' she urged, '… It is a woman's duty to use all the means in her power to beautify and preserve her complexion.'

Home-made Remedies and Secret Make-up

Without the concealing aid of make-up, a fine complexion became even more important and was an indicator of youth, health and social standing.

Fair skin and a lily-white hand were de rigueur to distinguish a lady from the weather-beaten working classes. Tight lacing certainly helped in achieving a refined pallor and fashion journals advised never stepping outside without a protective armoury of accessories including gloves, bonnet, veil and parasol.

Domestic manuals included innumerable home-made recipes for whitening and preserving the skin. *The Toilette of Health* (1834) recommended a concoction of bitter almonds, oxymurite of quicksilver and sal ammoniac to remove suntan; suggested distilled juice from green pineapples 'to take away wrinkles' and pimpernel water to blanch the complexion. 'Fresh beans, boiled in water, crushed and applied as a poultice on the freckles, will produce excellent effects,' advised another household guide, adding that if this didn't work, freckles 'the despair of blondes', could be dabbed with an uncomfortable sounding mixture of turpentine and camphor. 'Greasy skins are benefited by washing in the juice of fresh cucumbers. Equally good is the water in which spinach flowers have been boiled. The juice of strawberries is still better.'

Women plundered the garden for herbs and flowers and fed their faces from the kitchen. Lola Montez reports how Parisian ladies bound their faces with strips of raw beef as a night-time moisturiser whilst Spanish women squeezed orange juice in their eyes to add a bit of sparkle: 'The operation is a little painful for a moment, but there is no doubt that it does cleanse the eye, and impart to it temporarily, a remarkable brightness,' she reassured readers.

Overt skin painting and shop-bought cosmetics were frowned upon, 'A violently rouged woman is always a disgusting sight and … excessive use of powder is also a vulgar trick,' insists Lola, but she adds a little vegetable rouge was acceptable when 'used with the most delicate taste and discretion' along with a dusting of the finest powder, although 'the lady should be especially careful that sufficient is not left upon the face to be noticeable to the eye of a gentleman.' Basically as long as make-up was virtually imperceptible, worn only in the evening, and preferably home-made,

JULY 2, 1887   THE ILLUSTRATED LONDON NEWS   11

THE BEAUTY OF THE SKIN
ENHANCED BY

Ladies will find this delightful and refreshing

TOILET POWDER

invaluable as an application for the skin, reducing a too ruddy complexion and heightening a pallid skin to a beautiful tint. Its application absorbs all moisture, and induces that coolness and comfort to the skin so desirable in the ball-room, theatre, or in the open air.

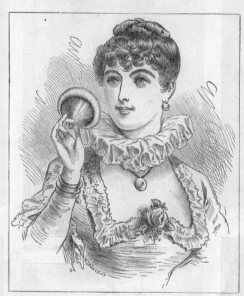

PRICE **1/-** PER BOX.

Per post, free from observation, 1/3.

IN THREE TINTS:
BLANCHE, for fair skins;
NATURELLE, for darker complexions;
AND
RACHEL, for use by artificial light.

OF ALL CHEMISTS AND PERFUMERS.

SOLE WHOLESALE AGENTS:

R. HOVENDEN & SONS,
31 & 32, BERNERS-STREET, W.;
AND
91–95, CITY-ROAD. LONDON, E.C.

POUDRE D'AMOUR.
PREPARED BY PICARD FRÈRES.

1887 advertisement for Poudre d'Amour by Picard Frères.

you could get away with a little bit of it. *The Toilette of Health* suggested darkening the eyelashes and brows with elderberry juice, burnt cork or burnt cloves; recommended rouging the cheeks by rubbing them with a red ribbon soaked in brandy, and included DIY recipes for vegetable rouge (made from cochineal), simple face-powders and even a scarlet lip salve, tinted with alkanet root.

Criminal Cosmetics

One of the reasons women were encouraged to produce their own cosmetics is that with no legislation in place, it was impossible to assess the ingredients and the potential after-effects of manufactured products.

'We venture to pronounce every cosmetic, the composition of which is kept a secret from the public, to be false and fraudulent, and that mercury and lead are their leading constituents,' declared *The Toilette of Health* firmly.'As a general rule it is prudent to avoid the use of all cosmetics the composition of which is a secret or unknown,' agreed the *Encyclopaedia of Domestic Economy* (1855). 'Resulting to artificial methods incurs two serious risks,' expanded the *Cornhill Magazine* in 1863,'the risk of injury to health, and the risk of being found out and despised.' And of course the risk of being conned.

That same year Mme Rachel (born Sarah Rachel Russell, former old clothes dealer and alleged prostitute's madam) opened a salon in London's elegant Bond Street, with the phrase 'Beautiful

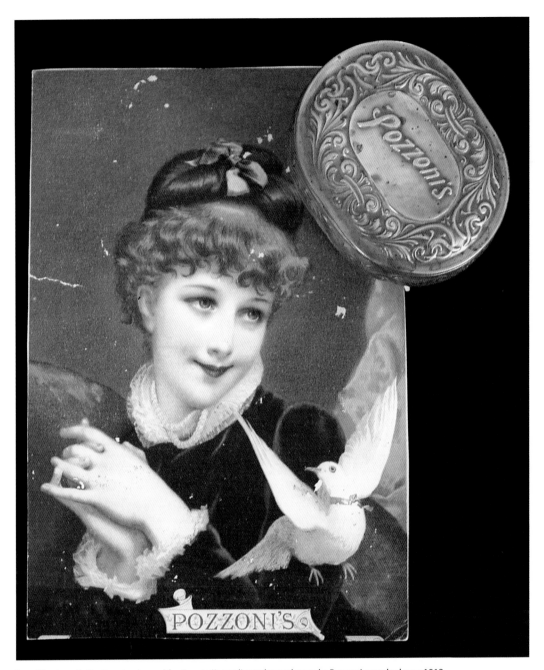

Late Nineteenth Century trade card for Pozzoni's medicated powder and a Pozzoni powder box c.1912.

for Ever' inscribed over the door. Claiming to be cosmetic advisor to the Sultana of Turkey and Empress Eugenie, she offered a range of over sixty exotic products including Alabaster liquid, Circassian Bloom (a favourite Victorian euphemism for blusher), Armenian Powder and Magnetic Rock Dew Water, which carried from the Sahara desert by 'swift dromedaries' in order to preserve its freshness, would eradicate all signs of ageing.

Heavily veiled society ladies visited the salon for private consultations and expensive treatments ranging from face enamelling at twenty guineas a time, to courses of 'Royal Arabian Baths' costing hundreds of pounds. These miraculous oriental washes were eventually revealed to consist of little more than bran and water mixed in the backyard, and in 1878 their imaginative supplier was sentenced to five years' for defrauding and blackmailing her embarrassed lady clients. Mme Rachel died in prison, but her name outlived her. Rachel became the term used to describe a standard face-powder colour, which according to an 1887 advertisement for Picard Frère's 'Poudre d'Amour', was best used in artificial light.

The Birth of Mass-Produced Beauty – The People's Stores

More respectable manufacturers sought to distance themselves from such rogue traders, by stressing the safety of their products: Beetham's Glycerine and Cucumber 'Ensures soft white skin. Beware of imitations, many of which are poisonous.' Pozzoni's Medicated Complexion Powder 'Contains no Lime, White Lead or Arsenic … Warranted Perfectly Harmless.'

Whilst make-up might have been beyond the pale there was no shame attached to buying skin and hair improvers. With growing urbanisation in the second half of the Nineteenth Century women were increasingly turning to shop-bought remedies and it wasn't just well-born ladies.

Improved quality of manufacture and enthusiastic advertising certainly fuelled the creation of this new mass-produced beauty industry, but another important ingredient was the discovery of a new (or at least untapped) group of consumers.

In the USA, the local drugstore, which became a fixture of every small town and the 'Five and Dime' store, pioneered by Frank Winfield Woolworth, who opened his first shop in Utica, New York in 1878, helped make beauty products available to a wider and less well-off sector of the population. In Britain, the pharmacy business was revolutionised and democratised by Boots.

In 1849 John Boot began selling herbal remedies from a small store in Goose Gate, Nottingham, but it was his son who transformed Boots from just another local pharmacy servicing a middle and upper class clientele into 'Chemists to the Nation'. Taking over in the 1870s, Jesse Boot (1850-1931), a devout Methodist, realised that the new growth area was the better-off working classes, who in the booming Victorian economy, could stretch to a few modest purchases. By buying in bulk and increasing his volume of sales, Jesse was able to reduce prices, undercutting more middle class chemists by as much as fifty per cent. Victorian doctors had a monopoly on making up prescriptions and their charges were often beyond the means of the poor who resorted to cheap quack remedies. After the monopoly was lifted in 1880 Jesse employed his own pharmacist who, much to the fury of rival establishments, dispensed half price prescriptions.

Jesse changed the branding of the shop to 'The People's Store', then to 'Boots Cash Chemist', emphasising its affordability. Special offers were advertised by a bell-ringer touring the streets of Nottingham; the store stayed open till 9pm most weekdays and 11pm on Saturdays so that customers could shop after work. Unsurprisingly, business flourished. By the turn of the century Boots had 180 shops, rising to 560 by 1914. 'Perfumery and Toilet Requisites' were an immensely popular line, dispensing affordable beauty to the masses and Boots Cash Chemists' Cold Cream became a British best-seller.

Buying a perfect skin

Skincare was a booming industry. Cold cream was a long established cooling moisturiser. The earliest known recipe for this emollient of fats and water is attributed to Galen, the celebrated Second Century Greek physician and in France cold cream is still known as cerat de Galien (Galen's Cream). By the late Nineteenth Century cold cream was produced by everybody from provincial chemists to the smartest Bond Street perfumers, who supplied their upper class clientele with 'delicately fragranced' preparations.

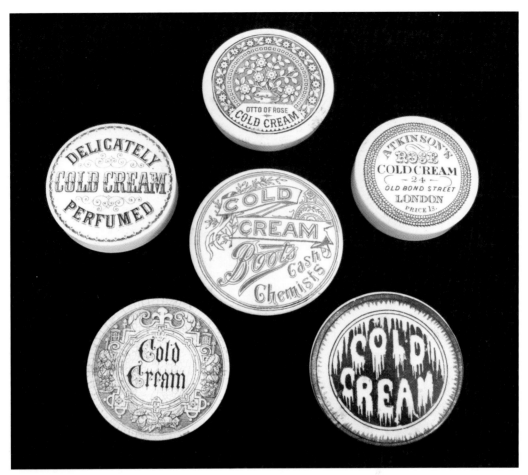

A collection of Victorian Cold Cream pot lids.

Complexion whiteners were another Victorian favourite and from Beetham's Cucumber and Glycerine to Aspinall's Neigeline ('Absolutely Non Poisonous' promised advertisements) there was a huge range of mass-produced potions designed to blanch the skin, and remove spots, freckles and socially inferior signs of sunburn.

New skincare remedies came from America. In the 1840s, Theron T. Pond discovered that the native American Oneida people, based in the New York area, were using a concoction of boiled witch hazel to salve burns and wounds. Pond collaborated with the tribe's medicine man and c.1846 launched Pond's Extract (initially known as Golden Treasure). By the 1880s Pond's had expanded their line to include toilet cream, lipsalve and soap, and although advertisements stressed their healing properties women were increasingly turning to Pond's for beauty.

At the same time as Pond's were developing their business Robert A. Cheeseborough, a young New York chemist, visited an oil well in Pennsylvania, hoping to benefit from this burgeoning new industry. One of the by-products of oil extraction was 'rod wax', a sticky petroleum residue that clogged up drilling rigs. Cheeseborough noticed the oil workers rubbing it on their hands to heal cuts and burns. He took away a sample, refined and processed it, and in 1872 patented Vaseline petroleum jelly. The name was allegedly derived from the German word for water, *wasser*, and the Greek word for oil, *elaion*, but whatever its origins, it was certainly a better choice than rod wax.

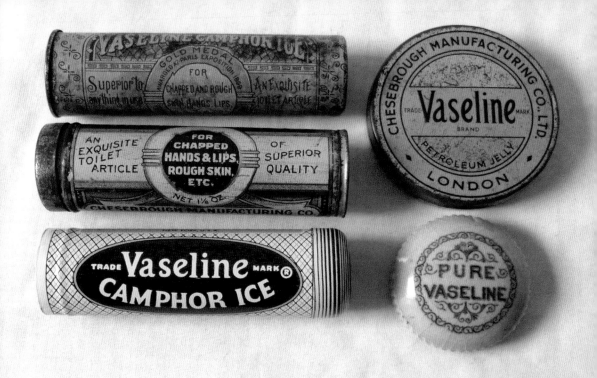

Above: A collection of vintage Vaseline containers dating from the late Nineteenth Century to the 1950s.

Right: Harriet Hubbard Ayer's Moth and Freckle lotion. Moth was a Nineteenth Century term for blotches or liver spots.

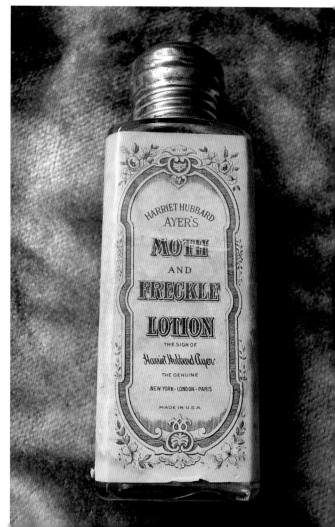

Like Pond's Extract, Vaseline was initially sold as a medical product, but ladies began using it as a moisturiser, hair oil and lipgloss, and soon to the company's delight, petroleum jelly was appearing on every dressing table. 'It will keep the skin clearer, softer and smoother than any cosmetic ever invented, and will preserve the youthful beauty and freshness of the healthy complexion,' claimed a Vaseline ad for 1881; announcing new cosmetic lines including Pomade Vaseline (for the hair), Vaseline Cold Cream, and Vaseline Camphor Ice (for pimples and blotches).

It wasn't just businessmen who were profiting from a booming beauty industry. American socialite Harriet Hubbard Ayer (1849-1903) survived bankruptcy, divorce, the death of a daughter in the great Chicago fire of 1871 and even incarceration in a lunatic asylum (not to mention depression and drug addiction) to reinvent herself as newspaper beauty columnist and successful manufacturer of cosmetic preparations. Her Recamier creams (allegedly made to a recipe used by Mme Recamier, the famous Napoleonic beauty), could it was claimed instantly remove spots, freckles and blackheads. Persistent use would prevent a bad complexion which, Mrs Ayer assured readers of the *New York Times* in 1887 'has been the original cause of more estrangements between lovers and husbands and wives than any other thing.'

The Fragrant Lady

Face creams were not the only acceptable Victorian beauty products. In a world of uncertain hygiene, perfume was another requisite. Although Mum, said to be the world's first commercial deodorant, was developed in Philadelphia in 1888, it wasn't until the 1920s that deodorants became commonplace. Scent was needed both to create and cover up smells, but fragrances had to be chosen with care. 'Above all, avoid strong, coarse perfumes and remember that if a woman's temper can be told from her handwriting, her good taste and breeding may easily be ascertained by the perfume she wears,' warned Eugene Rimmel in his *Book of Perfumes* (1867). 'Whilst a lady charms us with the delicate aetherial fragrance she sheds around her, aspiring vulgarity will as surely betray itself by a mouchoir redolent of common perfumes.' 'Vulgar' and 'common' were two Victorian buzzwords guaranteed to provoke fear in the hearts of the newly emerging middle

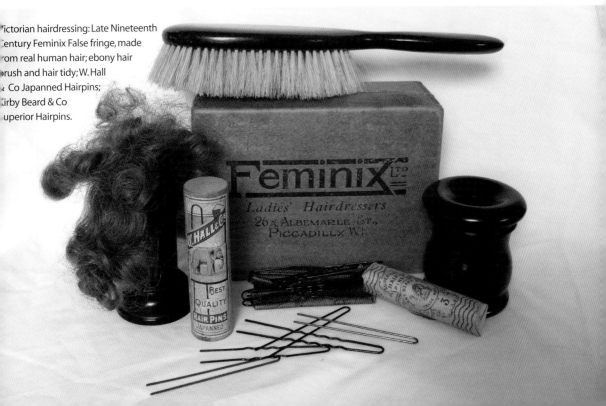

Victorian hairdressing: Late Nineteenth Century Feminix False fringe, made from real human hair; ebony hair brush and hair tidy; W. Hall & Co Japanned Hairpins; Kirby Beard & Co superior Hairpins.

classes. Etiquette manuals advised ladies to stick to gentle and natural fragrances: eau de cologne, rose, violet, lavender and orris root. 'A refined woman will always reject odours which are too strong,' advised Baroness Staffe in *The Lady's Dressing Room* (1893). The only place pungency was allowed was in the bottle of smelling salts or vinaigrette that corseted ladies (prone to fainting) kept close to hand.

Crowning Glory

Another popular line produced by fashionable London perfumers such as Atkinson's and Grossmith was fragranced hair oil.

Luxuriant locks were integral to feminine charm and lack of make-up was compensated for by extravagant hair care. Beauty manuals recommended brushing the hair for ten minutes minimum, up to four times a day. Dressing table sets included a 'hair tidy' (a screw-top container with a hole in the lid) which was used as a receptacle for what must have been a considerable amount of hair from the brush. This could then be combed out and transformed into additional hairpieces (familiarly known as 'rats') – cheaper and a much better colour match than buying in the false

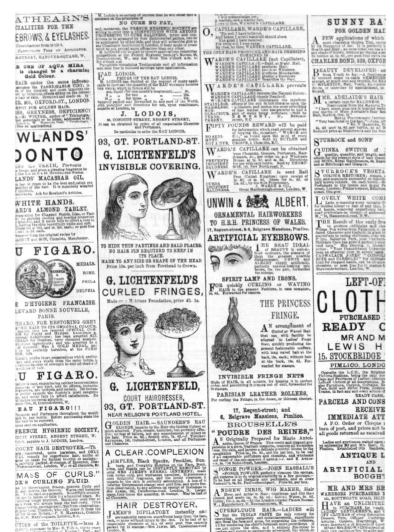

Advertisements for wigs, hair pieces and even artificial eyebrows from *The Queen, The Lady's Newspaper*, 1880.

ringlets and pads necessary to create the more complicated Victorian and Edwardian hairstyles. 'For evening, dinner hair ought to be dressed in four rolls either side or finished off behind with a Marie Antoinette chignon, frizzed very much,' advised *The Englishwoman's Domestic Magazine* in 1863.

Wigs

If your hair didn't 'frizz' naturally, or was simply too thin for fashionable hairstyles, you could try a wig. By 1865 Britain was the leading purchaser of human hair from France, importing (according to *The Times* newspaper), 11,954 ready-made chignons, along with enough loose hair to produce 7,000 more. Hairdressers offered everything from curled fringes to full on wigs – euphemistically referred to as 'invisible coverings'. For the most follically-challenged ladies, Unwin and Albert 'Ornamental Hairworkers to HRH Princess of Wales' even supplied artificial eyebrows at fifteen shillings the pair.

Wigs (to say nothing of stick-on eyebrows) were not without their problems. Cartoonists illustrated them falling off, and as contemporary photographs demonstrate, all too often false hairpieces were anything but invisible – sitting on top of the head like a small furry animal. Baroness Staffe (ever the purveyor of doom-laden beauty news) warned that false hair could transmit the skin diseases of its original owner and added that hair cut from a living person (although expensive) would last for only two years, after which it needed to be renewed; while hair taken from dead people, 'never sold by hairdressers who value their reputation' was almost impossible to curl.

Curlers and Crimpers

The alternatives to a wig were frizzing your own hair with curling papers and pins which, as the Baroness observed, was an uncomfortable process, or using curling tongs.

Despite the risks of burning (again stressed by the Baroness) curling and crimping irons were standard dressing table items. Various new models were introduced in the Victorian and Edwardian periods and if you came up with a good design, it could make your fortune.

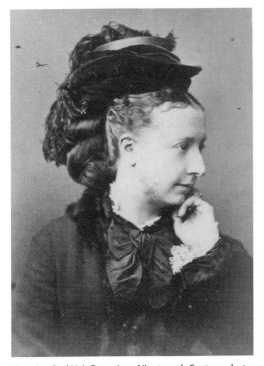 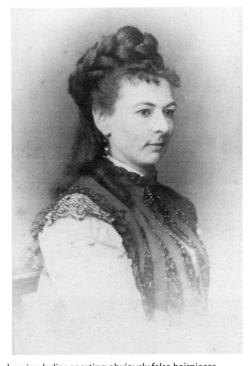

Victorian Bad Hair Day – Late Nineteenth Century photographs showing ladies sporting obviously false hairpieces.

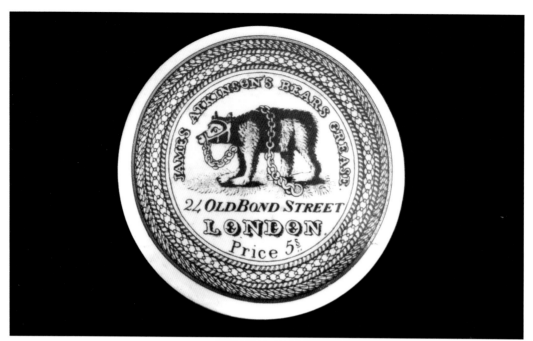

Victorian-style pot lid for James Atkinson's Bears Grease.

The French coiffeur Marcel Grateau, son of a poor stonemason, began his career cleaning the windows of a Parisian hairdresser for few centimes. He migrated inside the salon, worked his way up and in 1872, devised a new type of curved curling tongue that created a natural ripple rather than a harsh crimp. 'L'Ondulation Marcel', the 'Marcel wave' became a huge hit. Marcel's hair tongs sold across the world and by 1897 Marcel himself was a millionaire and retired to a château in the French countryside.

German Barber Karl Nessler (1872–1951), immigrated to London where he developed the permanent wave machine, using sodium hydroxide (a strong alkali) and electricity. After several unsuccessful attempts and twice burning off his wife's hair, the first public demonstration of permanent waving took place at his Oxford Street salon in 1906. Using the trade name Charles Nestle, Nessler ran a successful business curling the heads of the aristocracy until World War I, when he was interned as an enemy alien. He fled to New York in 1915. Nessler established salons across the USA; he also developed a permanent wave machine for home use that cost only $15 and sold in its thousands.

Pomades and Hair Oils

Elaborate Victorian hairstyles, and the drying effects of curling, stimulated demand for pomades, hair oils and bandolines (gum-containing setting lotions).

Perfumed bear's grease, an expensive product, was used by both men and women to promote hair growth. Brown bears were the favourite source (resulting in the decimation of the ursine population of Russia); reindeer and buffalo were sometimes substituted and according to contemporary crime reports, London dog thieves occasionally stole older, less valuable canines for boiling down into counterfeit bear's grease. Small wonder that by the last quarter of the Nineteenth Century vegetal lotions – made from coconut, palm and olive oils – had largely taken over.

Rowland's Macassar oil – produced by the London firm of A. Rowland & Sons from the early Nineteenth Century onwards – was one of the best known. Said to be made from plants native

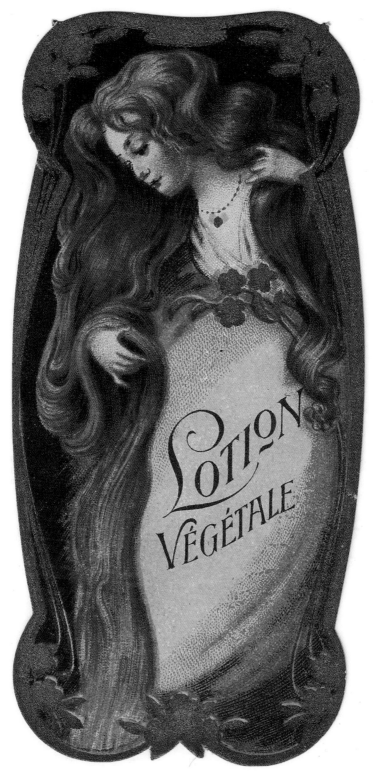

Lotion Végétale label c.1900.

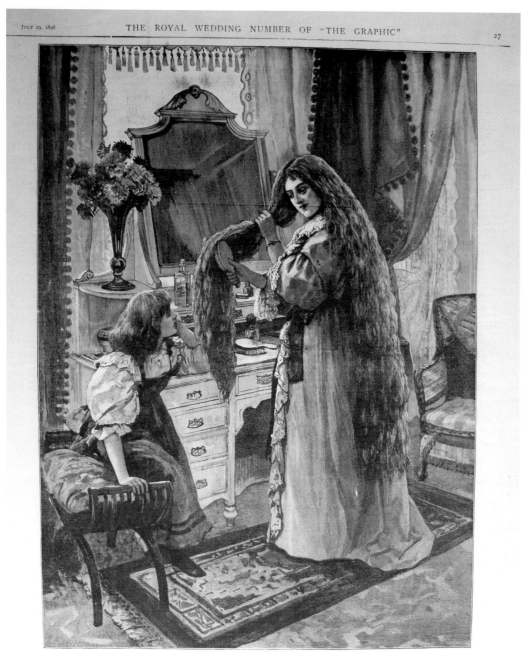

Advertisement for Harlene Hair restorer, 1896.

to Macassar in Indonesia, it claimed to promote the most luxuriant tresses, while preventing everything from baldness to greyness. What it certainly did was leave greasy marks on the furniture – hence the introduction of the antimacassar (a little cloth designed to protect the chair back).

Other Victorian and Edwardian best-sellers included Mrs Allen's Worlds Hair Restorer; Koko (said to stimulate the brain, along with the hair); Rexall Tonic 'Promotes Hair Health – Your Money Back If It Doesn't'; and Edwards' Harlene 'the great hair producer and restorer'. Harlene advertisements featured women with scarily long tresses and, like most other lotions, mysteriously promised to return the hair to its natural colour without using dye. 'When her third husband died, her hair turned quite gold from grief,' quipped Oscar Wilde in *The Picture of Dorian Gray* (1891). Colouring the hair was commonplace, but as with using cosmetics, you would be unlikely to admit to it and by many hair dye still wasn't considered quite proper, or entirely safe.

'The number of bald women increases every day,' lamented Baroness Staffe. 'This state of things is attributed to the curling irons, which have been too much used; to the wigs; to the false hair, which has caused the real to fall out … There is very likely some truth in all this; but in my opinion it is to the dyes, above all, that the evil is due.'

Victorian newspapers were filled with advertisements for hair restorers, pomades, dyes, but curiously to modern eyes, the one product missing from a seemingly endless list of lotions and potions was shampoo, which in the Nineteenth Century had a slightly different meaning.

First recorded in the English language in 1762, the word shampoo derives from the Hindi verb champo, meaning to press or massage. The pioneer of shampooing in Britain was a remarkable Bengali soldier, Sake Dean Mahomet (1759-1851). Born in Patnar, Mahomet served in the English East India Company Bengal Army, before emigrating to Ireland where in 1786, he published *The Travels of Dean Mahomet*, the first ever book to be written by an Indian in English. Moving to London, he opened the Hindustani Coffee House in 1809 – the first ever Indian-owned restaurant in Britain – then when that went bankrupt, he moved to Brighton where he established the country's first shampooing vapour baths. Mahomet's medicated massage with Indian oils was said to cure everything from gout to baldness, and he was appointed 'Shampooing Surgeon' to both King George IV and William IV. Though shampooing (head rubbing) was practised by barbers, cream shampoo (as we know it today) did not really emerge until the 1930s when Procter and Gamble launched Drene; claimed to be the first synthetic (non soap) shampoo. In the Nineteenth Century the most common form of hair wash was soap and water, contributing still further to the expansion of the Victorian soap business.

Cleanliness is next to Godliness – Soap and Water

'Cleanliness is, indeed, next to Godliness,' preached John Wesley, founder of the Methodist movement in the Eighteenth Century. It wasn't until the Victorian period, however, thanks to improved sewerage and water supplies in Britain, the opening of the first publicly funded baths and wash houses, and in 1852 the repeal of the tax on soap, that cleanliness could at last become a more achievable earthly reality.

Every etiquette guide stressed that washing and personal hygiene were the very cornerstones of beauty, virtue and domestic harmony. 'Friction is never to be neglected by those who would shine in the courts of beauty,' advised Lola Montez. 'To my thinking one must be clean before one can be really good. Dirt and religion do not blend,' added Harriet Hubbard Ayer, who recommended a minimum of one bath a day (preferably two) in order to avoid 'the sin of dowdiness', which could cost a woman both her good looks and her husband. As a divorcee herself marital rifts were a subject that Mrs Ayer returned to frequently in her beauty advice.

Soap manufacturers flourished in this new climate of cleanliness. In 1885 William Hesketh Lever launched Sunlight Soap, which containing palm and vegetable oil lathered more easily than traditional household soaps made from tallow and animal fats. Orders flooded in and after only two years the company was selling 450 tonnes of Sunlight Soap a week, laying the foundations for the mighty Unilever Corporation (est. 1930). Popular Victorian brands subsequently purchased by Lever included Erasmic and Vinolia soap, which was later supplied to first class passengers on the maiden voyage of the *Titanic*.

In the USA, William Colgate opened a starch, soap and candle factory in New York in 1806 (toothpaste wasn't launched by the firm until the 1870s). William Procter and James Gamble also began a company producing soap and candles in 1837. Though the arrival of the electric light bulb eventually killed off the candle side of the business their soap went from strength to strength. During the American Civil war Procter and Gamble were contracted to supply soap to the Union Army and in 1879 they launched their famous Ivory brand. The soap was named from the Bible 'all thy garments smell of myrrh, and aloes, and cassia, out of the ivory palaces, whereby they have made thee glad' (Psalm 45) and promoted with two major selling points: its purity and the fact that it floated in the bath. From Lever's carbolic Lifebuoy soap (1894) 'Cleans, Disinfects … robs life's perilous voyage of the dangers of infection' to the gentle Palmolive, introduced by the B.J.Johnson Co. in Milwaukee in 1898 and containing palm and olive oil, many long-lasting brands were created in the second half of the Nineteenth Century. However one Victorian success story was in fact far older.

In 1789 London hairdresser Andrew Pears began experimenting to create a new soap that would be kind to the complexion. It was refined to remove irritants, perfumed with English flowers and above all see-through, stressing its purity. Pears' transparent bars were a hit, and he was soon forced to sign each packet, with 'my own quill' in order to distinguish his product from cheap copies. Pears was a successful small business, trading to a predominantly upper class clientele, until the second half of the Nineteenth Century when Thomas J. Barratt married Andrew's great-granddaughter.

Often referred to as the father of modern advertising Barratt had a genius for promotion. In the 1880s French ten centime pieces could be used in Britain where they were worth one penny. Barratt imported a quarter of a million coins from France and since there was no law prohibiting the defacing of foreign currency, he stamped 'Pears' on each one and released them into circulation. Suddenly the name of the company was in every pocket, forcing a new Act of Parliament which made foreign coins illegal tender. Other less controversial coups included publishing *Pears Annual*, which offered fiction and fine quality frameable prints for only sixpence; launching *Pears Shilling Cyclopaedia* – which unlike traditional encyclopaediae was priced and written for the general public – and the purchase of Sir John Everett Millais' painting *Bubbles* (1886), for promotional purposes.

Barratt reproduced the picture in advertisements, adding a cake of Pears transparent soap underneath the feet of the curly headed, bubble-blowing boy (Millais' grandson). Sir John Everett Millais, 1st Baronet, President of the Royal Academy and pillar of the art establishment, was accused of prostituting his art and his family in order to sell soap. *Bubbles* became one of the most famous paintings in the world, Pears was associated with art and culture in the public imagination and business boomed.

Barratt was also a pioneer of celebrity promotion. In the 1880s opera singer Adelina Patti and Lillie Langtry – actress, famous beauty and close friend of Edward, Prince of Wales – both appeared in Pears advertisements, claiming that all you needed to achieve perfect looks and matchless complexion was a tablet of Pears transparent soap. But looking at the enhanced features of these and other stage beauties in contemporary photographs and illustrations clearly this wasn't always the case. As the Victorian Period gave way to the Edwardian Belle Epoque not only were actresses becoming more socially acceptable but so was a little bit of make-up.

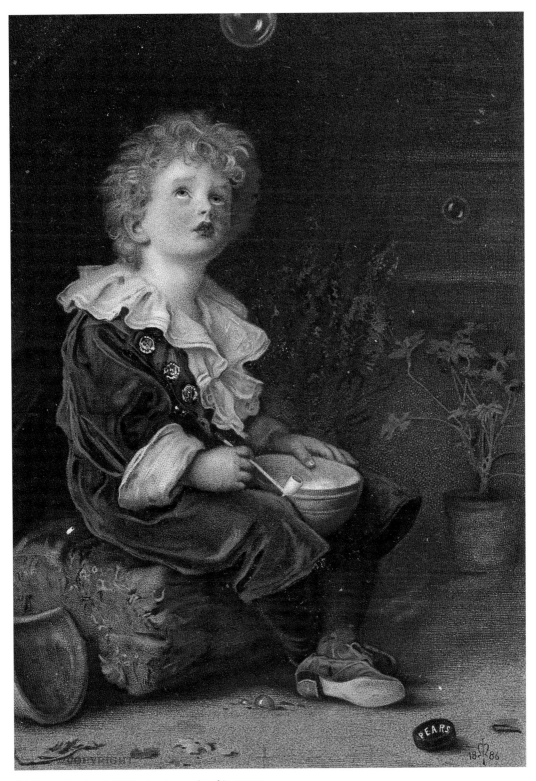

Bubbles postcard, early 1900s, showing a cake of Pears soap.

CHAPTER THREE

Actresses, Mistresses, and Suffragettes

Beauty in the Belle Epoque, 1890–1914

'NAY, BUT IT IS useless to protest. Artifice must queen it once more in the town. The Victorian era comes to its end and the day of *sancta simplicitas* is quite ended … For Behold! Are not men rattling the dice-box and ladies dipping their fingers in the rouge-pot?' demanded Max Beerbohm in his satirical essay *A Defence of Cosmetics* (1894).

From the sinuous curves of Art Nouveau fashions, to Oscar Wilde's *Dorian Gray* selling his soul for eternal handsome youth, there was a different attitude to beauty at the fin de siecle. Writing in the first issue of *The Yellow Book*, (the journal that epitomised modern day decadence) Beerbohm portrayed a society where Victorian values had been overturned and a pretty face had nothing to do with virtue and everything to do with make-up. 'Within the last five years the trade of the makers of cosmetics has increased immoderately – twenty-fold, so one of these makers has said to me. We need but walk down any modish street and peer … under the bonnet of any woman we meet, to see over how wide a kingdom rouge reigns … Fashion has made Jezebel surrender her monopoly of the rouge-pot … For the era of rouge is upon us.'

PETER ROBINSON, LTD., 252 to 264, REGENT ST., W.

"MARAVEL" GUINEA CORSET.

Perfect in cut and style, quite low in the bust, and deep over the hips; the breast darts being graduated into the waist, give comfort and freedom to the figure. Made in best quality White Coutille, and boned Real Whalebone, with Silk Stocking Suspenders attached, **Price 21s.** Same style in Black Sateen, **Price 23s. 6d.**

Edwardian advertisement for the Maravel Corset, c.1900.

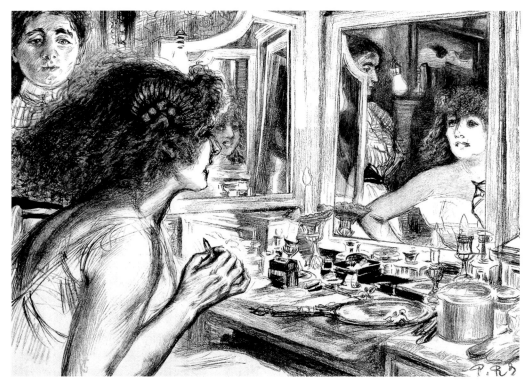

Sarah Bernhardt in her dressing room, from *The Graphic* newspaper 1894.

In the 'naughty nineties', a decade that kicked of with cancan girls revealing their all at the newly opened Moulin Rouge in Paris and in which theatre and music hall became more popular than ever before, performers were certainly influential in promoting a more open use of beauty products.

Theatrical Make-up

The one area where cosmetics had flourished in the Nineteenth Century was the stage, thanks largely to improvements in theatrical lighting. Gas illumination was introduced in the early 1800s; by the middle of the century limelight (created by shining a gas torch at a solid block of lime) had made it possible to spotlight artists, and the 1880s saw the first completely electrified theatres.

Performers who found themselves literally in the limelight needed better cosmetics than the crude powdered chalk and white paint that had sufficed for candles and oil lamps. The invention of greasepaint is attributed to German actor Carl Baudin, from the Leipziger Stadt Theatre, who mixed lard with zinc white, yellow ochre and vermillion to create a flesh-coloured paste. Greasepaint in stick form was first sold commercially in the 1870s by the Wagnerian opera singer Ludwig Leichner (1836-1912), who set up a stage make-up company in Berlin. According to an 1877 theatrical make-up guide the round sticks cost 6d each and were numbered from light to dark. No.1, the lightest flesh colour, was for 'ladies with a delicate complexion'; no.1½ was for ladies playing 'chambermaid parts'; no.4 was 'a dark ruddy colour suitable for soldiers, sailors, countrymen etc.', whilst no.7 was 'for mulattoes'. In Paris the perfumer Alexander Napoleon Bourjois was supplying theatrical cosmetics at the same period and Bourjois' distinctive little round boxes of 'pastel joues' (claimed by the company to be the world's first powder blusher) gradually spread beyond the theatrical community, as society ladies followed the lead of actresses.

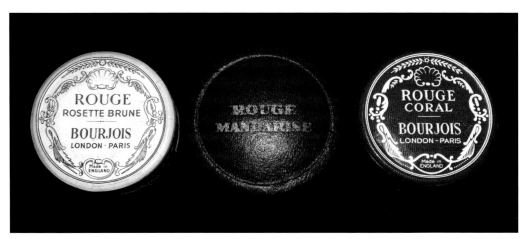

Vintage boxes of Bourjois rouge.

Stage Beauties

Far from being dismissed as Jezebels, performers were increasingly portrayed as celebrity style icons. Thanks to improvements in printing and photography their image was disseminated in every form from song sheets to picture post cards, which when introduced at the turn of the century stimulated a massive collecting craze. The popular press followed their every move. In 1894 *The Graphic* newspaper showed the divine Sarah Bernhardt making-up at her dressing table, surrounded by cosmetic accessories. Magazines reported actresses' beauty tips and women imitated their clothes and hairstyles. Mrs Langtry – the famous Jersey Lily – was responsible for a plethora of new fashions ranging from the Langtry bustle (a curious contraption of hinged metal bands that concertinaed when a lady needed to sit down, and sprang back into place when she stood up again) to a figure-hugging knitted outfit, inspired by fisherman's clothing on her native Channel island, and named in her honour; the Jersey.

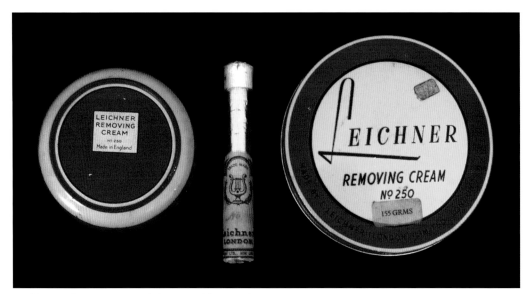

A collection of vintage Twentieth Century Leichner products.

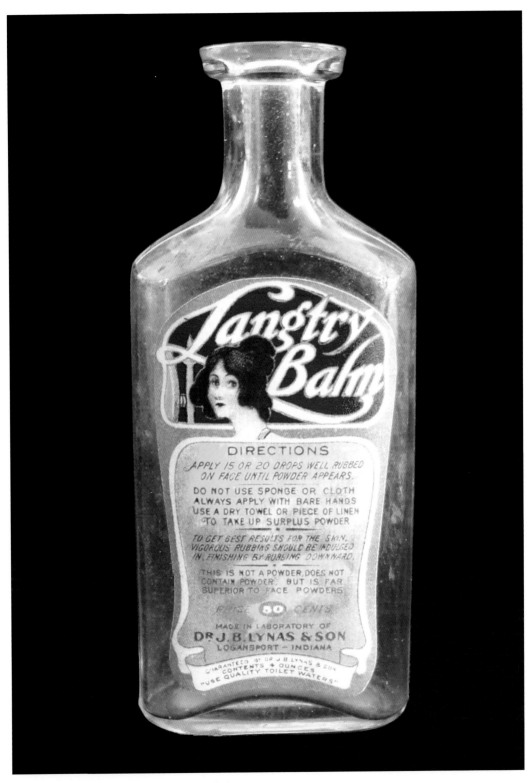

Langtry Balm liquid face powder, early Twentieth Century.

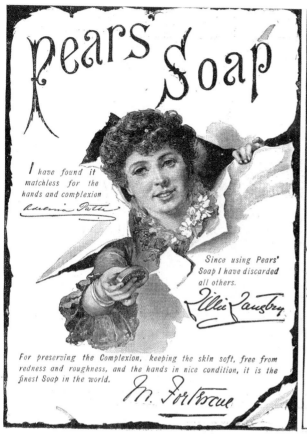

Lillie Langtry advertisement for Pears soap dating from the 1880s.

Cosmetic companies cashed in on actresses' popularity. Theatre programmes were a favourite advertising venue for beauty products and manufacturers paid performers to promote their wares. Sarah Bernhardt powdered her face and exposed her magnificently snowy cleavage in a famous poster for La Diaphane poudre de riz (1890). She also endorsed lotions for Harriet Hubbard Ayer, who owed much of her success to using actresses in advertisements including Lillian Russell, Lillie Langtry and Adelina Patti. Patti 'The Queen of Song' was almost as remarkable for her business acumen as her voice. At the height of her fame in America she demanded $5,000 to be paid into her hands in cash before each performance (no money, no singing) and she lent her name to so many products from corsets to face creams that she gained the soubriquet 'Testimonial Patti'. But for manufacturers of beauty products endorsements from the most famous beauties of the day were almost worth their weight in gold. Lilly Langtry is said have been paid £132 for endorsing Pears Soap – exactly what she weighed in pounds – and allowed her name to be used on face powders and skin balms.

Women wanted to look like actresses; men wanted to look at actresses, and in the changing moral climate of the fin de siecle – Jezebels or not – their social standing improved. The fun-loving Prince of Wales surrounded himself with a very different circle from Queen Victoria: the 'frivolous, selfish and pleasure-seeking rich' moaned his unamused mother. Edward's chosen companions included American millionaires, Jewish financiers, and British nouveaux riche: who all helped finance the Prince's luxury life-style whilst at the same time, to a certain extent, democratising the monarchy.

Royal Mistresses

You didn't need to be well born to enter the charmed royal circle but you did have to be wealthy or pretty. Edward enjoyed liaisons with various stage beauties including Lillie Langtry and Sarah Bernhardt. At his Coronation in 1901, a pew (dubbed 'the King's loose box') was reserved in Westminster Abbey for mistresses past and present lead by the lovely Mrs Alice Keppel, his most famous companion and with curious serendipity, great-grandmother to Camilla, Duchess of Cornwall; wife of the current Prince of Wales.

Behaviour at Edward's court was also more flexible than during Victoria and Albert's uxorious rule. As long as you were married, discreet and didn't divorce, infidelity was perfectly acceptable. Mrs Keppel was received everywhere by everybody, even Queen Alexandra, and the royal affair was an open secret ('King's Cross,' directed Alice as she climbed into a hansom cab en route to the station.'Not with you, Ma'am,' was the driver's alleged reply).

In aristocratic circles at least new freedoms also influenced attitudes to cosmetics. While unmarried girls were expected be unpainted, married women had more licence. Queen Alexandra was among the first great ladies of the Edwardian era to openly wear powder and rouge. Mrs Keppel was equally fastidious about her beauty. She creamed her face every night and slept on a silk pillow in order to preserve her complexion. Personal effects discovered in a bank vault many years after her death included an enamelled Fabergé compact – opening to reveal a gold-mounted swansdown powder puff, still smelling faintly of her scented face powder. The same strong box, filled with gifts from the King, also revealed a number of Fabergé cigarette cases. Edward was a prodigious smoker, consuming an average of twelve cigars and twenty cigarettes a day. Alice also smoked, matching her jewelled cases to her dress, and using a long and elegant cigarette holder.

It was unusual for a women to smoke in public, but one of the advantages of being part of the 'Marlborough set' (Edward's inner circle) was that middle class conventions could be flouted. One of the more bizarre aristocratic cosmetic fashions of the day was a vogue for tattooing. As a young man, Edward had a Jerusalem Cross tattooed on his arm during a visit to the Holy Land in 1862. Twenty years later when his sons, the Duke of Clarence and the Duke of York (later King George V) were in Japan, both had dragons tattooed on their arms. It wasn't just men. In 1903, whilst on a trip to the East, Edith, Marchioness of Londonderry had a coiled snake tattooed on her leg. Lady Randolph Churchill, mother of Winston, was rumoured to have a snake round her wrist, concealed by a bangle. Leading London tattooists of the 1900s included George Burchett (Britain's most famous tattoo artist) and Sutherland MacDonald (based in fashionable Jermyn Street) both of whom attracted an upper class clientele. In addition to providing images Edwardian tattoo studios also offered a 'permanent tinting' service for the more daring society lady; tattooing cheeks pink, darkening eyebrows and outlining the lips.

Powder & Rouge

Permanent or otherwise, for the upper classes at least, make-up and cosmetic treatments were becoming a little more available. In 1886 Mrs Francis Hemming started an exclusive London salon to sell her Cyclax cosmetics (ladies still preferred to enter secretly by the back door) and beauty parlours became increasingly popular in America.

Face powder was in general use and came in decorative cardboard and metal containers. Packaging reassured women that the contents were safe and ladylike to use: Parker's face powder 'Harmless, Beautifying and Refreshing'; Lablache face powder 'Used and endorsed by the most Refined Ladies in Private and Public Life'. As cosmetic historian Richard Corson observes, although few respectable women in the early 1900s would have openly admitted to using rouge 'clearly many of them did – or wanted to.' In 1907 *Vogue* recommended 'La Belle Coquette', a very natural looking cream rouge from France which came concealed in a Limoges porcelain bonbon box pretty enough to satisfy 'the most dainty of her sex' and discreet enough

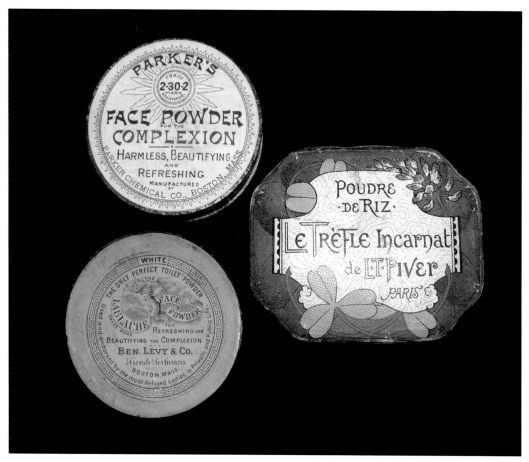

Face powder boxes early Twentieth Century: Parker's Face Powder; Lablache Face Powder; Le Trèfle Incarnat de Piver.

not to look like a rouge pot. Selfridges, which opened in Oxford Street in 1909, became the first British department store to put cosmetics and perfumes on open display. Rather than being hidden under the counter beauty products were placed right by the front entrance, so that customers would be instantly greeted by sweet and seductive fragrances – a position they have occupied ever since.

With the end of the Nineteenth Century attitudes were indeed changing and not just when it came to rouge. The expansion of shops and the creation of new department stores such as Selfridges, the introduction of telephone exchanges in 1880s and above all the invention of the typewriter created a wealth of new jobs for middle-class young women – even if they were poorly paid and expected to retire upon marriage.

Thanks to another technological innovation, women also had more freedom of movement. Initially it had been considered unsuitable and gynaecologically dangerous for ladies to ride one of the new safety bicycles that replaced the penny-farthing. But with the development of the drop frame bicycle one major obstruction, the cross bar, was removed. Women took up cycling and left their chaperones standing.

Thanks in part to the bicycle and to increased female involvement in sport (tennis, archery, golf, croquet) a new outfit emerged – a simple fitted skirt and jacket inspired by the riding habit and by men's suits. By the 1900s the tailor-made costume was worn by everybody from royalty to

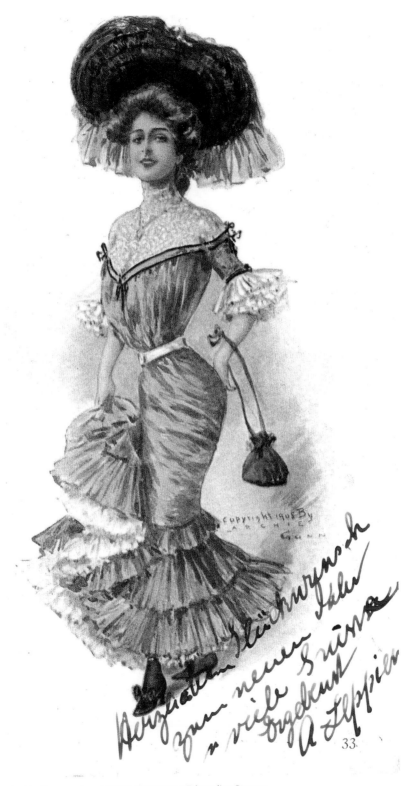

Archie Gunn postcard (1905) showing an Edwardian Beauty.

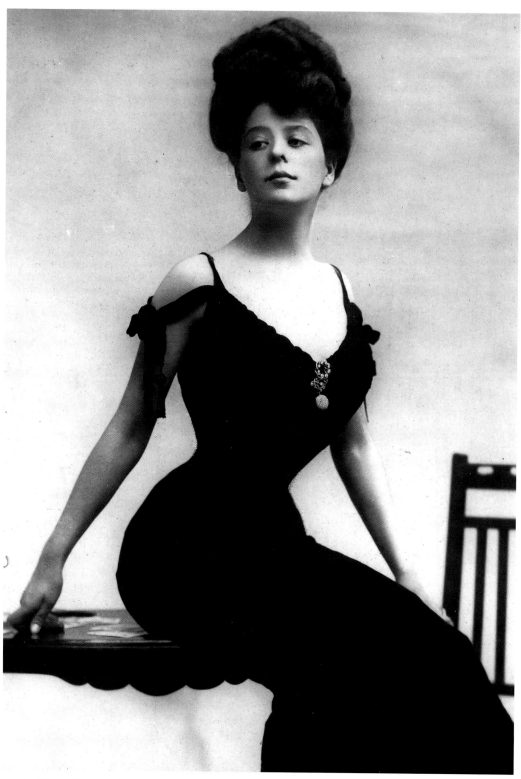

Camille Clifford 'Gibson Girl' postcard – early 1900s.

typists and whereas the Victorian lady was shaped like a bell, the Edwardian silhouette was very different.

The Gibson Girl

In the 1890s American graphic artist Charles Dana Gibson (1867-1944) drew a new female archetype: a lively, feminine young woman, with an ample bosom, a wasp waist, and a curvaceous, sticking out bottom, shown off by a long straight skirt. The S-shaped Gibson girl with her abundant hair piled high on her pretty head, became the Edwardian ideal.

Camille Clifford won a magazine contest to find a real life version of the Gibson girl and, from 1902 until her fairy-tale marriage into the British peerage in 1906, she enjoyed a successful stage career. Her acting and singing might not have been up to much but audiences flocked to the theatre to watch her do the 'Gibson Walk' in a daring, skin-tight black velvet dress and her remarkable hourglass figure was reproduced in countless photographic postcards.

This was an age that prized womanly curves. Edward's mistresses were notable for their generous figures (as indeed was Edward himself whose spherical shape gained him the unflattering nickname Tum-Tum) but unlike the king, ladies were expected to go in as well as out.

Even if she didn't have to wear a crinoline and could whiz along on her bicycle, the Edwardian woman was just as imprisoned by fashion as her mid-Victorian predecessor. The Gibson look could only be achieved with vicious underwear and a new corset developed by Frenchwoman Mme Gaches-Saurraute in 1900, which starting low on the bust and extending well down over the hips, twisted the body into the requisite S-shape. The waist was drawn in as tight as possible – Camille Clifford's measured eighteen inches. The abdomen was pulled backwards pushing out the bottom. The bust was thrust forward with a boned bodice (precursor of the bra) that created a vast, overhanging mono-bosom, reminiscent of a pouting pigeon.

If your chest was unfashionably small, the bodice could be supplemented with padding or you could try massaging in 'Princess Bust Cream Food', which prepared by 'an eminent French Chemist', promised to create a plump, full rounded bosom, particularly when applied with Dr Fuller's Princess Bust Developer, a curious implement resembling a toilet plunger.

A lady's neck was ideally long and slim, set off by a high collar or a broad jewelled choker – the necklace popularised by Queen Alexandra who used it to conceal an unsightly scrofula scar. The neck was made to look even more swanlike in contrast with a huge pompadour hair style, (built up with numerous false hair pieces) and surmounted by an even more enormous hat, decorated with flowers, feathers, and perhaps a complete stuffed bird. One of the reasons for the founding of the RSPB, which received its royal charter in 1904, was to protect the rare grebe from being slaughtered for the sake of millinery.

Hats were anchored to the hair with decorative hatpins: twelve-inch long, viciously sharp and potentially dangerous. Ladies were banned from wearing hatpins with unprotected ends on omnibuses. Suffragettes appearing in court were allowed to keep their decorated hats, but hatpins were confiscated in case they used them as weapons.

Suffragette Style

In *A Defence of Cosmetics* (subsequently reprinted under the title *The Pervasion of Rouge*) Max Beerbohm observed that, alongside the rouged artificial beauties lounging in front of their dressing tables in the 1890s, there was another new female role model. These 'horrific pioneers of womanhood who gad hither and thither' were already responsible for 'the invasion of the tennis courts and of the golf links, the seizure of the bicycle and of the typewriter', and their aim was 'the final victorious occupation' of the House of Commons. Beerbohm predicted that these agitating harridans would ultimately be defeated by the seductive power of cosmetics and fashion, which would distract ladies from rallying to their 'unbecoming' side.

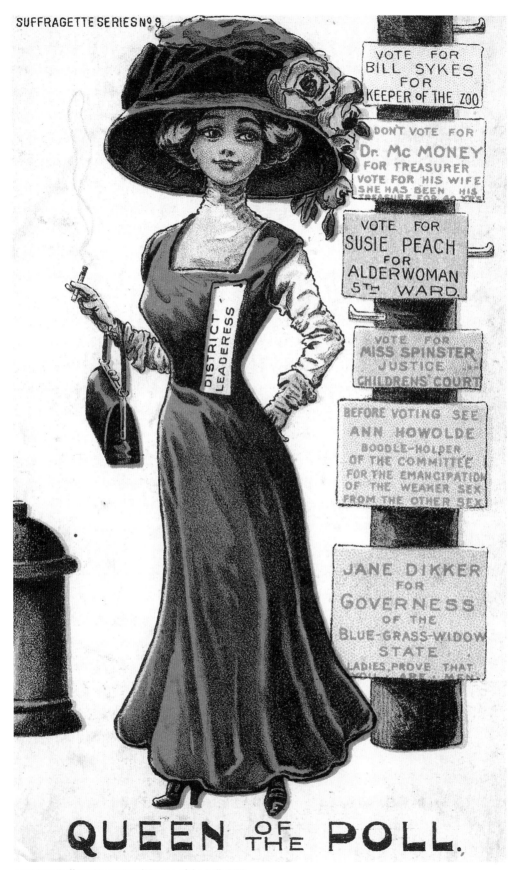

American Suffragette postcard 'Queen of the Poll', 1906.

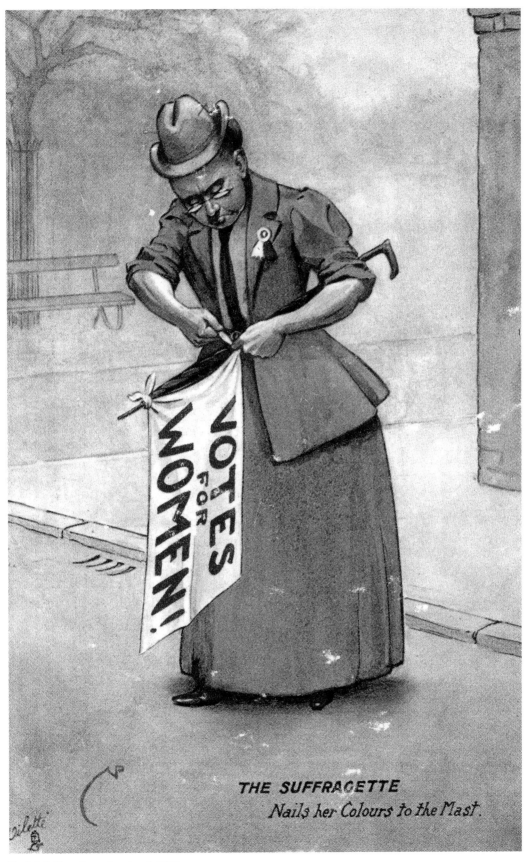

THE SUFFRAGETTE

Nails her Colours to the Mast.

English Suffragette postcard, early 1900s.

The popular press might have portrayed suffragettes as 'the Screaming Sisterhood', a rabble of butch spinsters in unflattering masculine clothing, but the reality was very different.

The women who fought so bitterly for the vote were the epitome of Edwardian feminine elegance. Wearing beautiful hats and snowy white dresses that set off their pretty purple, white and green suffragette sashes they dressed to confound the 'harridan' image; to create an attractive uniform, and to provide an extra frisson of surprise as a lovely lady in a picture hat lobbed a brick through a window. Derry and Toms, a smart department store in Kensington, advertised millinery in the *Votes for Women* newspaper and British suffragettes spent hours planning their outfits before rallies.

American campaigners for the vote not only dressed in the height of fashion but also made a political point of wearing make-up. On one famous demonstration in New York in 1912, all the ladies painted their mouths with shockingly bright red lipstick and Elizabeth Arden joined in the parade. Famous actress Lillian Russell, known as 'The American Beauty', was a prominent suffragist and at the same time launched her own cosmetics brand in 1914. 'In placing my own toilet preparations on the market I was largely influenced by a desire to help woman kind generally as I have helped myself,' she assured purchasers of the Lillian Russell Beauty Box containing 'My own Purity Face Powder' and even 'My own Lip Rouge'.

Whilst the explicit intention of the suffragists was Votes for Women the implicit message was that whether they were 'New Women' cycling in bloomers and sensible shoes, or elegant ladies in big hats and bright lipstick, women should be free to choose what they wanted to look like and who they wanted to be. Campaigners weren't defeated by the 'pervasion of rouge', in fact many of them embraced it. But for the right to vote and the freedom to apply make-up in public without censure it would take a World War.

On the Turn of the Century Dressing table

Victorian and Edwardian ladies might not have much make-up, but dressing tables were anything but empty. Elaborate vanity sets were produced in a wide range of materials from china to tortoiseshell. Decorated silver was a favourite choice for wedding presents – plain bone or ebony provided an affordable, everyday alternative.

Alongside the basic trio – hand mirror and two hairbrushes – came innumerable accessories, many concerning the laborious process of getting dressed. Shoehorns, clothes brushes and a bonnet whisk were standard additions. Buttonhooks were provided in different sizes for boots, underwear, gloves etc., all of which came with a wealth of fiddly fastenings. Women squeezed into gloves so tight that they could only be put on with the assistance of a glove stretcher and a glove powderer – the long necked shaker designed to reach right down into the fingers.

A dainty, lily-white hand was the mark of a lady. Nails were polished with chamois leather and could be coloured a natural looking pink with rose tinted oil or paste. In the 1900s *Vogue* reported on the new fashion for transparent liquid polishes that were painted on with a camel hair brush. In 1911 American firm Northam Warren launched Cutex cuticle remover, the foundation of a mighty nail care empire. Small manicure implements, with silver, ivory or mother of peal handles came in boxed sets; sometimes also including needlework tools – uniting vanity items with virtuous industry.

Powder was one of the few acceptable cosmetics and came in three main colours: white, natural and Rachel. At home dressing table sets had matching powder boxes, and toilet powder was applied with lambswool and swansdown powder puffs or a rabbit's foot. Though no lady would be seen powdering her nose at the dinner table, by the 1900s discreet powder compacts and miniature mirrors could be worn suspended from chatelaines. In 1903, American *Vogue* recommended Papier Poudré. The little books with their powdered pages could be easily hidden in a handbag and 'Powder applied from these leaflets has the advantage of other forms in that it does not soil the corsage when being applied.' Patches or beauty spots popular in the Eighteenth Century remained

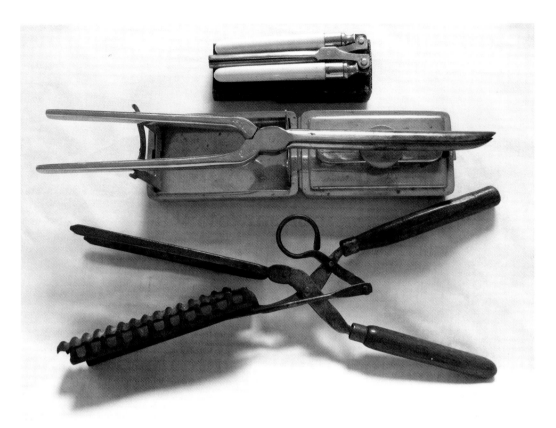

Wooden handled hair crimper; Marcel tongs on portable spirit lamp heater; bone-handled folding tongs for travelling, with box.

in occasional use during the Victorian period, providing a useful way of covering up an embarrassing spot and like compacts, little mirrored patch boxes could be slipped into a reticule.

The Nineteenth Century saw the development of mass produced skin care. Cold cream was purchased in white earthenware pots, the same as those used for bear's grease, tooth paste and countless food products from potted meat to fish paste. Lids were typically under glaze printed in black and chemists could either buy a generic cold cream design from the potteries, or have their own name and details transferred onto the lid. Skin whiteners and hair remedies were supplied in disposable glass bottles and, as with pot lids, surviving examples have often been rescued from Victorian rubbish dumps.

Much of the dressing table was given over to hair care. Tall holders were provided for hatpins and small pin trays for hairpins, which were purchased in paper wraps and cardboard tubes. Hairpin manufacture flourished in the Victorian period, mostly centered around Birmingham, heart of the metal industry. Hairpins were initially smooth and straight but in 1856 J. Edridge patented corrugated shapes: 'To cause such pins to take firmer hold in the hair.' Well-known manufacturers of the period include Kirby, Beard & Co., suppliers to Queen Victoria, whose name is immortalised in the term Kirby grip; registered in 1926 to describe a shorter, sprung hair grip that, like the American bobby pin, was created to deal with the new bobbed hairstyles.

There were different designs for curling tongs. Crimping irons produced elaborate waves and for travelling there were folding irons and portable spirit lamps which could also be used at home to heat tongs on the dressing table.

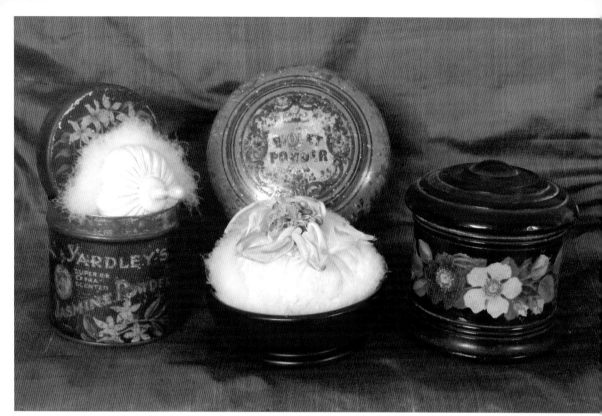

Late Nineteenth Century Yardley Jasmine Powder tin; wooden container for Violet Powder; swansdown powder puff; ebony powder box decorated with roses.

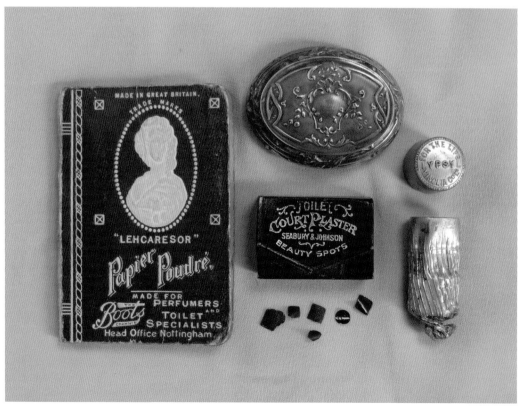

Lehcaresor Papier Poudré made for Boots; Joilet Court Plaster Beauty Spots – Seabury & Johnson – late Nineteenth Century; Art Nouveau metal patch/powder box with mirrored interior c.1900; Lyspy for the lips, Vinolia Co. USA, c.1910.

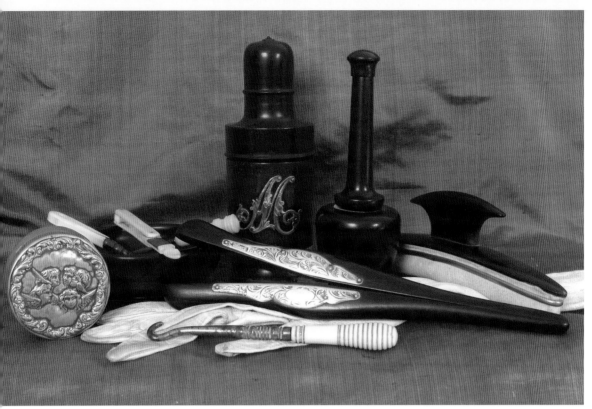

Silver trinket box, decorated with Reynolds' angels; ebony bowl, perfume bottle holder with silver M, glove powderer, nail buffer and silver-mounted glove stretcher; bone and ivory handled manicure implements and button hook – late Nineteenth Century.

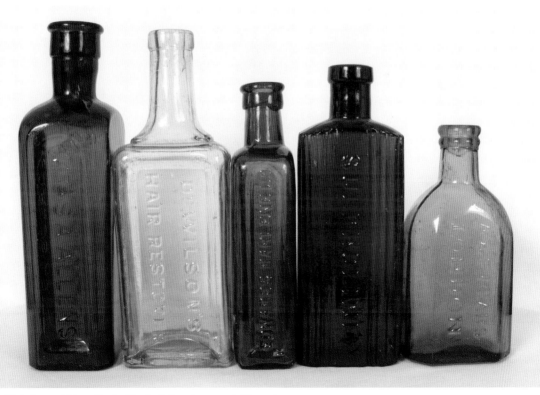

Victorian and Edwardian bottles for hair restorers and skin washes.

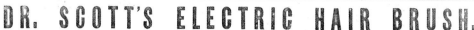

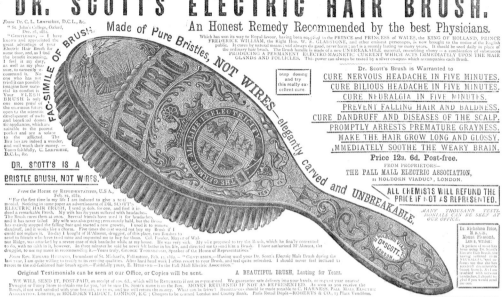

Victorian advertisement for Dr Scott's Electric hairbrush, 1882.

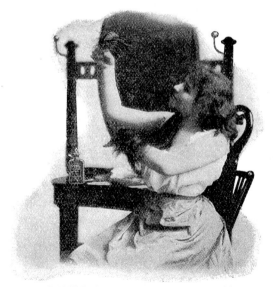

American advertisement for the Coke Dandruff Cure, 1899.

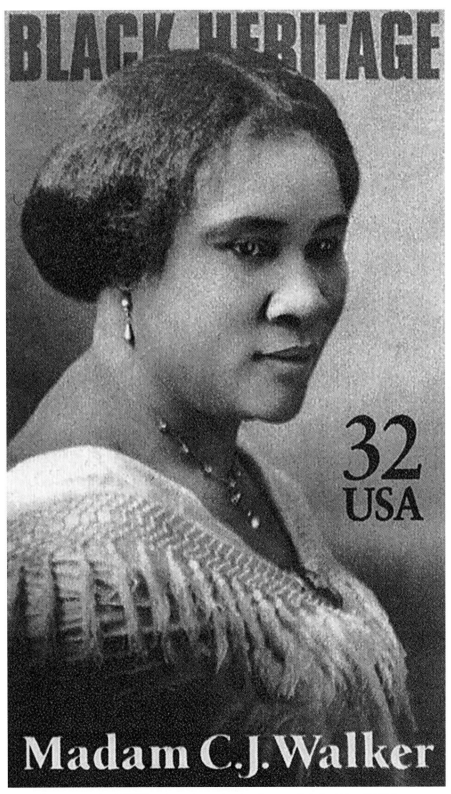

BLACK HERITAGE

32 USA

Madam C.J. Walker

Commemorative 1998 US postage stamp showing the smooth-haired Mme C.J. Walker.

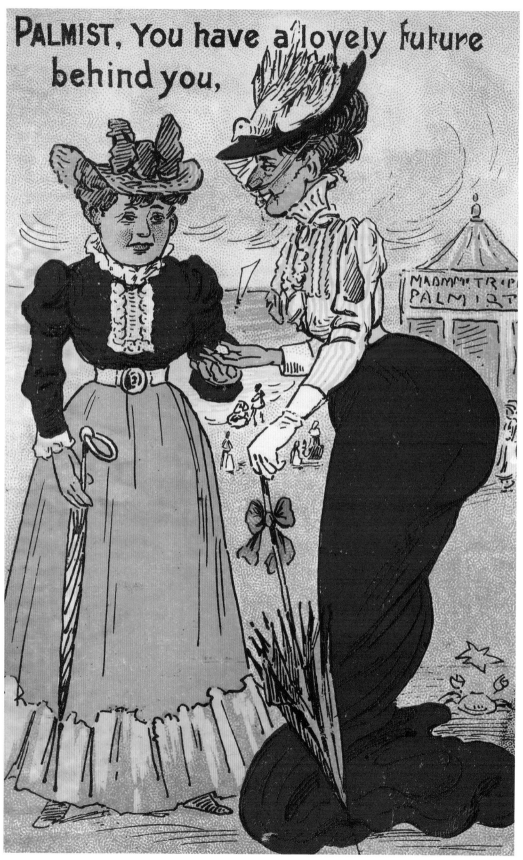

Comic postcard satirising Edwardian fashion, early 1900s.

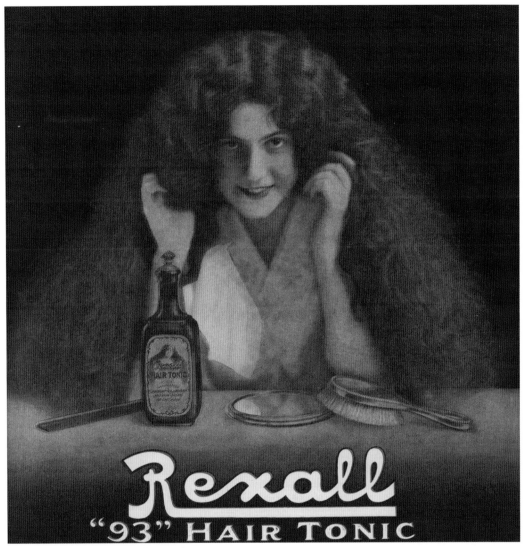

Rexall hair tonic advertisement from 1911.

Hairbrushes too came in various styles – long-handled brushes were preferred by women; for men oval 'military' brushes were supplied in pairs. Famous brands of the period included long-established suppliers (William Kent founded his famous London brush company in 1777) and innovative new firms. In 1885 British engineer Mason Pearson invented an automatic brush-boring machine to speed up the manufacturing process and also developed a 'pneumatic' rubber-cushion to support the bristles. In 1906 American entrepreneur Alfred C. Fuller borrowed $375 to set up the Fuller Brush Company in Boston, selling hair and household brushes. Fuller not only produced a high-quality product that came with a lifetime guarantee but was also one of the pioneers of door-to-door salesmanship. The Fuller Brush man became a familiar figure across the US, (the teenage Billy Graham honed his preaching skills as a Fuller representative) and by 1919 the company was turning over $1 million.

Kent, Mason Pearson and Fuller are still well-known names today. Less long-lasting however was the Victorian vogue for 'galvanic' hairbrushes, which promised to restore hair colour and remove all 'rheumatic and neuralgic affections of the head'. Dr Scott's Electric Hairbrush, patented in 1881, had magnets embedded in the handle and would, according to the advertisements, cure everything from baldness to constipation.

Hair pomades and restorers made equally extravagant claims and quack scalp remedies contained everything from mercury to cocaine. Whatever the attendant dangers, hair related products were probably the most popular cosmetic purchases of the day. The industry boomed and not just with a white, middle class clientele.

One of the most remarkable success stories of the 1900s was Madam C. J. Walker (1867-1919). Born Sarah Breedlove to freed slaves in poverty stricken Louisiana, Sarah Breedlove was orphaned at seven, married at fourteen, widowed at twenty and worked as a washerwoman and a cook before in her thirties developing a home-made scalp conditioner to treat her own thinning hair. In 1906 she married Charles Joseph Walker and that same year launched Madam C. J. Walker's 'Wonderful Hair Grower'. She went on to manufacture a range of hair and cosmetic products sold by and to African-American Women, pioneering a powerful new market. At its height her company employed 3,000 people and by the time of her death in 1919 Madam C. J. Walker was America's wealthiest African-American woman; said to be the first ever US female, black or white to become a self-made millionaire.

As women of different classes and colours embraced new freedoms at the dawn of the Twentieth Century manufacturers recognised that there were huge profits to be made from the beauty business, and never again would a lady's dressing table be comparatively free from make-up.

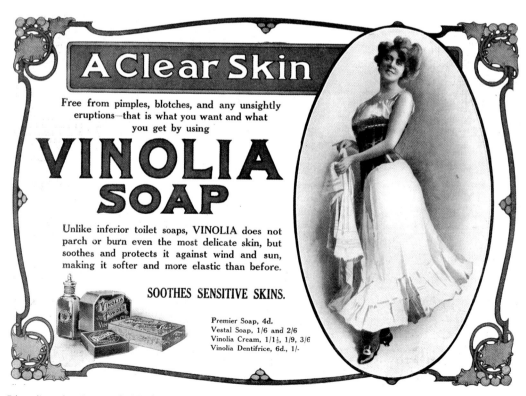

Edwardian advertisement for Vinolia soap.

CHAPTER FOUR

Put on a Pretty Face

Beauty in the 1920s

WORLD WAR I changed everything, including the looks and lives of women. As men went to the Front, so women replaced them in the workplace. 'It is quite impossible to keep pace with all the new incarnations of women in war-time – bus-conductress, ticket-collector, lift-girl, club waitress, post-woman, bank clerk, motor-driver, farm-labourer, guide, munition maker … whenever he sees one of these new citizens … Mr Punch is proud and delighted,' approved *Punch* magazine in June 1916.

In their land girl britches and factory overalls, many women were literally wearing the trousers for the first time, earning an income and a new sense of independence. 'The war revolutionised the industrial position of women – it found them serfs and left them free,' explained Mrs Millicent Fawcett, president of the National Union of Women's Suffrage Societies.

Partly in recognition of their war work, and following the pre-war efforts of the suffragettes, parliament granted the vote to women over thirty in 1918. The following year the Sex Disqualification Removal Act made it illegal to exclude women from jobs because of their sex and, in theory at least, they could now become solicitors, barristers and magistrates. Women across the USA gained suffrage in 1920 and in 1928 the female voting age in Britain was reduced to twenty-one the same as for men. But turning up at a polling station wasn't the only sign of post-war equality in the roaring twenties.

FLAPPER FASHIONS – Is it a girl, is it a boy?

'Men and women are becoming every year more indistinguishable,' observed *Vogue* in 1922 as a new generation of jazz dancing, cigarette smoking and cocktail drinking flappers bobbed their hair, shortened their skirts and threw away their whalebone corsets.

The dominant female look of the roaring twenties was the androgynous 'La Garconne' – a name inspired by the sexually emancipated heroine of Victor Margueritte's 1922 eponymous and scandalous novel. 'Slenderness today is the first requirement of beauty,' advised American *Vogue* (Feb.1925). 'Buxom … is anathema, and "boyish" takes its place.' Curling locks, trailing frocks and Edwardian curves were out. Like art deco design and American skyscrapers, the modern female silhouette was long, lean and geometric, 'flexible and tubular, like a section of boa constrictor … dressed in clothes that emphasised this serpentine slimness,' observed novelist Aldous Huxley, chronicler of the bright young things.

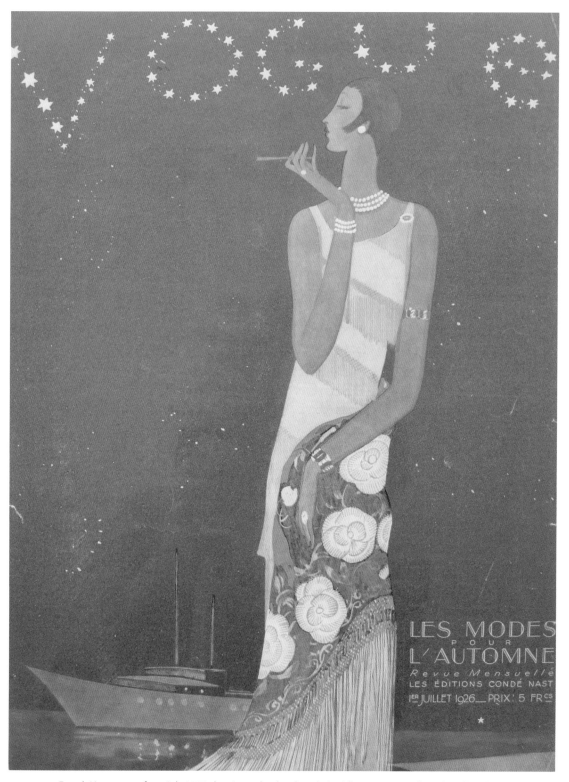

French *Vogue* cover from July 1926, showing a slender, short-haired flapper, wearing lipstick and smoking.

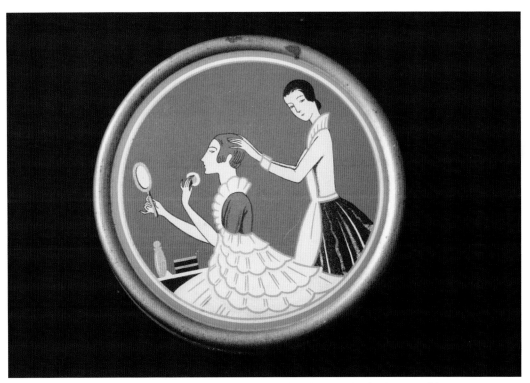

Richard Hudnut 'Three Flowers' Dusting Powder tin showing a lady and her maid at the dressing table, 1920s/30s.

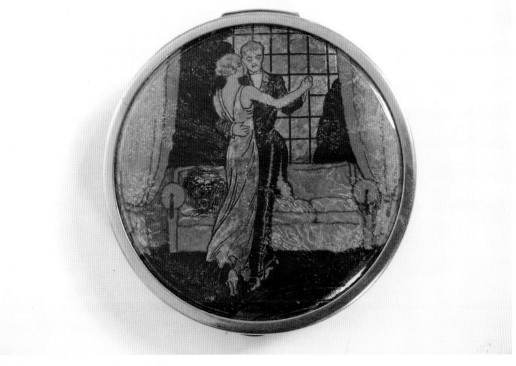

1920s foil compact showing couple dancing.

On the one hand this new look was extremely liberating. Short skirts were perfect for dancing the charleston and when French tennis star Suzanne Lenglen won Wimbledon in 1919 in a dress that daringly revealed her ankles and forearms, she ushered in a decade in which women could at last dress for (and as such play) sport. 'Anyone for tennis?' was a much more attractive proposition if you weren't going to trip over voluminous petticoats. *Vogue* featured women wearing trousers on the skiing slopes of St Moritz, and clinging one-piece jersey bathing costumes on the beaches of the Riviera. 'The modern girl is triumphant. She can wear anything she wants to wear,' trilled the magazine, but this new freedom came at a cost.

Shingled hair, streamlined clothing and increasingly revealed flesh meant that more emphasis was placed on the face and the body. The 1920s was the decade when cosmetic preparations and slimming aids truly came into their own, when home-made remedies were replaced by mass-production and beauty became a global business.

KEEP YOUNG AND BEAUTIFUL

'Keep young and beautiful, if you want to be loved,' warned a popular Hollywood song. The devastating number of casualties in World War 1 (3.1 million in Britain, 6.1 million in France), followed by the flu epidemic, had created a shortage of marriageable men and if you wanted to catch your man – and fit into the latest tubular fashions – you needed to look good.

In the first half of the 1920s ladies' magazines were filled with advertisements for face creams and body treatments. With colour illustrations often restricted to the front cover, copywriters painted pictures with words, using extensive copy and an aggressive approach: 'Have you a double chin? Or that ugly bagginess at the neck? Or the unsightly droop at the comer of the mouth?' demanded a typical advertisement for a beauty parlour.

Rather than stressing make-up and concealment, the main emphasis was on prevention, cure and what can occasionally seem like a good deal of physical punishment.

Writing in 1923 beauty specialist Eleanor Adair recommended smoothing wrinkles with moisturiser applied beneath the Ganesh chin strap and forehead strap to be worn whilst sleeping. American *Vogue* (1925) advertised slimming with Doctor Walters' rubber reducing garments: a corset for the hips, a rubber bandeau to reduce the bust and even rubber anklets, for those newly revealed legs. English *Vogue* suggested obtaining a more slender and youthful look with Viabella's 'radio-active mud treatment' and Clark's Thinning Bath Salts: 'Superfluous tissue literally melts through the pores.' If all else failed, the Norvic Body Binder, available from Boots, was a crêpe bandage that could be wound around the body to reduce unsightly bulges and was worn under clothing.

'Now that to be chic and to be slim have become synonymous we are all striving to reduce,' moaned the magazine, and with the rise of youthful streamlined fashions came the development of the beauty salons, founded by a new generation of female entrepreneurs most famously: Elizabeth Arden and Helena Rubinstein.

BEAUTY QUEENS

Small in stature (Elizabeth was 5ft 2, Helena 4ft 10), these two great rivals were big in character and huge in influence, pioneering the modern luxury beauty industry and introducing women to the daily ritual of cleansing, toning and moisturising, preferably with their own expensive products. 'Nothing that costs only a dollar is worth having,' declared Miss Arden.

Elizabeth Arden (d.1966) was born Florence Nightinghale Graham in Canada c.1881 though, like Miss Rubinstein, she was typically obscure both about her humble origins and the exact year: 'My dear, I've lied about it so often I can't even remember the date myself.'

In 1907 she moved to New York, working first for Eleanor Adair – where she learnt to apply the Ganesh strap – then opening a salon with Elizabeth Hubbard. When the partnership foundered after only six months Florence took over the business in 1910, changed her name to Elizabeth

Arden, and a legend was born. According to the Arden company history, by 1920 'over a hundred products were spelling out the Elizabeth Arden name in almost 600 permutations – more products than any other company in the world.' Salons were opened up in London and Paris, and in the 1930s it was said that there were three American names known in every corner of the globe: Singer Sewing Machines, Coca-Cola, and Elizabeth Arden.

'There is no reason for a woman to lose even one iota of her beauty,' insisted the redoubtable Miss Arden, who throughout her long life maintained a rigid routine of massage, exercise, manicures, pedicures, depilation, and countless other beauty treatments ranging from wax baths to electrical currents, all of which were available to her clients. Once behind the famous Red Door

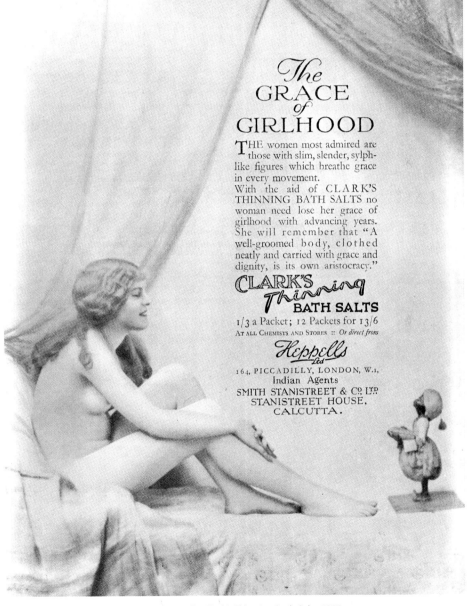

Advertisement for Clark's Thinning Bath Salts, 1920s.

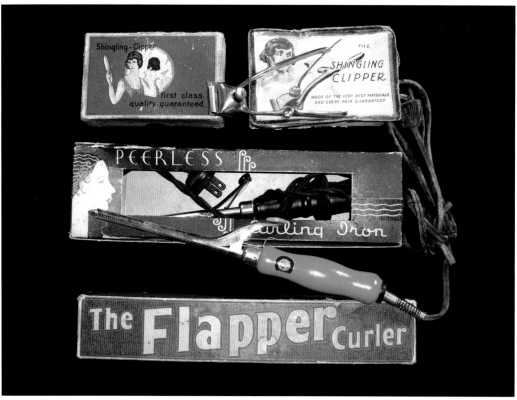

Curling irons and shingling clippers from the 1920–30s.

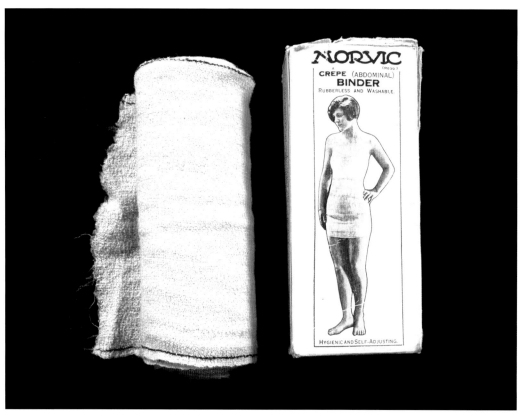

Norvic Body Binder – crêpe bandage, available from Boots, for getting rid of those unsightly bulges, 1920s.

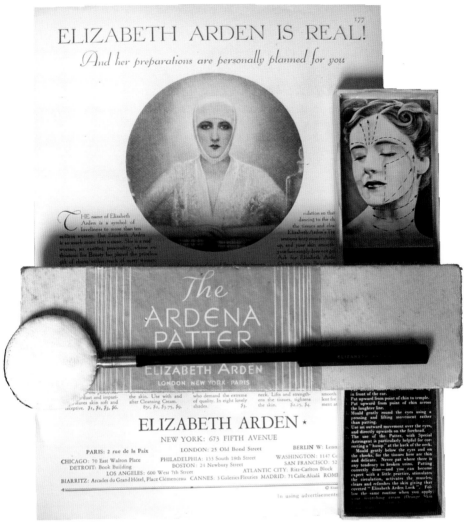

Elizabeth Arden advertisement, 1929, and vintage Elizabeth Arden Patter.

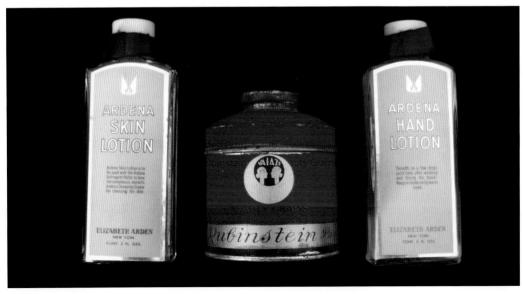

Ardena Skin and Hand Lotion, 1950s, Helena Rubinstein Valaze Beauty Grains, 1920s.

Helena Rubinstein Cosmetics Proclaim the Artist!

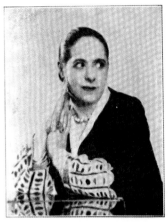

MME. HELENA RUBINSTEIN
World-Famed Beauty Scientist

THE secret of a successful facial ensemble? . . . Make-up that is as perfect in texture as in color . . . lipstick that lends satin smoothness as well as luscious tone . . . rouge you can blend with ease . . . powder so gossamer it becomes one with the skin . . .

Such are the cosmetics of Helena Rubinstein. For they are the creation of one who is artist as well as scientist . . . one who for years has divided her life between laboratory and atelier . . . studying constantly to bless all women with the wondrous coloring of immortal beauties.

When you touch the new Cubist Lipstick to your lips, when you bring the glow of Red Raspberry Rouge to your cheeks, when you clothe your skin with the gentle fragrant radiance that is Valaze Powder, then you realize the magic that lies in make-up.

For color, for texture, for staying quality, for wholesomeness, the cosmetic creations of Helena Rubinstein are unquestionably the finest in the world.

Ravishing Rouges

Valaze Rouges (compact or en creme) impart a luscious bloom that actually protects the skin! For daytime you will choose gay, piquant, youthful Red Raspberry, and for evening, Red Geranium, the vivid, the provocative. For the conservative woman there is the subtle Crushed Rose Leaves. 1.00 to 5.00.

The Magic Lipstick

Cubist Lipstick—Helena Rubinstein's newest cosmetic creation. Brings to the lips a softness, lustre and beauty rivalled only by the rare loveliness of its coloring. In two enchanting shades, Red Raspberry for day and Red Geranium for evening. To be chic one must have both. Smart enameled cases, Golden or Black. 1.00.

Water Lily Vanities

are masterpieces of the jeweler's craft! Enameled in Jet Black, Chinese Red, Jade Green or Golden. Double Compact 2.50, Golden 3.00. Single Compact 2.00, Golden 2.50.

Beautiful Eyes

Accent the Beauty of Your Eyes with Valaze Persian Eye-Black (Mascara)---instantly darkens the eyelashes, giving them an effect of silky, soft luxuriance. Wonderfully adherent, yet does not leave the lashes stiff or brittle. 1.00, 1.50.

Valaze Eye Shadow (Compact or Cream, in black, brown, green or blue). 1.00.

Valaze Eyelash Grower and Darkener promotes luxuriant growth of lashes and brows. 1.00, 1.50.

The Smart Woman's Beauty Treatment

Cleanse the skin with the luxurious Valaze Water Lily Cleansing Cream. Contains youth-renewing essences of water-lily buds (2.50). Revivify the face and eyes with the rare anti-wrinkle lotion, Valaze Extrait (2.50, 5.00, 10.00). Then wake the tissues with the unique rejuvenating stimulant, Valaze Eau Verte (3.00, 5.00, 10.00), and while the skin is tingling and responsive, pat in Valaze Emailline (1.75, 3.50, 6.00, 11.00), the bracing astringent massage cream. If muscles of face and throat droop, revitalize them with Valaze Georgine Lactee (3.00, 6.00, 11.00), a muscle tightener vital to sagging faces. A complete beauty treatment for the smart woman.

The Basis of a Chic Make-up

Before you apply your finishing touches, cleanse the skin with Water Lily Cleansing Cream— the exquisite youthifying cleanser, designed for the fastidious (2.50, 4.00, 7.50). Water Lily Foundation lends the skin a soft, alluring creaminess, makes rouge and powder doubly adherent, doubly flattering. An ideal powder foundation. 2.00. Now your skin is ready for—

A Powder Masterpiece

Valaze Powder. Clinging, exquisitely textured, subtly fragrant. In a rich variety of smart and enhancing shades. Novena for dry skin. Valaze for average and oily skin. 1.50, 3.00, 5.50.

It is essential that you visit Helena Rubinstein's Salons at this trying time of year, so that your beauty may present a harmony of perfection—skin, contour, eyes, hands and hair all exquisite. Here you will receive the last word in scientific beauty treatments and expert guidance on home treatments and make-up.

Helena Rubinstein advertisement, 1929.

that identified Arden salons across the world, you could have your face firmed with the Ardena 'patter', your fatty tissue broken down with the extremely vicious looking Francis Jordan roller and your posture and figure improved with her specially devised Corrective Exercises for Women.

'Beauty comes from within,' claimed Miss Arden, which didn't stop her or her rivals from offering a vast and profitable range of lotions and potions. Arden best-sellers of the twenties included Venetian creams and Ardena skin tonics, whilst the 1930s saw the invention of Arden's Eight Hour Cream, one of the most famous beauty products of all time, and which its creator used on the legs of her beloved race horses.

Helena Rubinstein's fortune began with her miracle Valaze skin food – a moisturiser made to a secret family recipe. Born in Krakow, Poland in 1872, she emigrated to Australia in 1896, with little more than some pretty dresses, a parasol and twelve pots of her mother's face cream to protect her from the Antipodean sunshine. 'My own skin was soft and fresh and remained so even in that terrible climate,' she remembered. Women asked her for the recipe and Helena set to work. Though advertisements claimed that Valaze skin food was imported from Europe at huge expense and 'compounded from rare herbs which only grow in the Carpathian mountains', as her biographer Lindy Woodhead points out, everything that Helena needed from lanolin, the oil from sheep's wool, to pine bark was ready available in the outback. Mme Rubinstein was mixing the ingredients herself, and adding the potent element of romance, without which a cream is little more than oil and water. Something else she manufactured quite brilliantly was the need for her creams. Rubinstein is said to have been the first beauty specialist to classify skin as dry, normal and oily. From one family recipe, she developed innumerable tailor-made products, which like Arden she took round the world, opening salons in Australia and Europe before moving to America in 1914, where, to Elizabeth's lifelong fury, she established a multi-million dollar business.

The genius of these two beauty queens was to mastermind the combination of luxury and perceived necessity that still makes skin care products so irresistible today. Cream wasn't a cosmetic but a 'skin food', you went to a salon for a 'treatment', and the salon itself occupied a new position midway between a beauty parlour and a medical centre. Roberta, famous model of the twenties, appeared in Arden advertisements with her beautiful head swathed in bandages. Madame Rubinstein called herself a 'cosmetic scientist' and was regularly photographed in a white lab coat, surrounded by bottles and test tubes. At her Valaze Salons she offered 'exclusive treatments … to remedy every possible beauty flaw' all administered 'under the supervision of a lady doctor'.

Miss Arden and Mme Rubinstein were the reigning beauty queens of the day but there were plenty of cosmetics princesses, opening salons, launching new must-have products, and supporting their wares with pseudo-scientific claims and enthusiastic if rather vague references to expert chemists and leading continental doctors.

In 1924, Phyllis Earle was offering a range of new products including Motor Cream, to protect the skin of the lady driver, Phantom Cream (a bleach for whitening the complexion) and Kemolite, a radio-active mask; all 'prepared in wonderfully equipped laboratories under the supervision of chemist-cosmeticians' and administered in 'surroundings of daintyness, restful charm and perfect hygienic cleanliness' at her 'Institut de Beaute' in central London.

Irrespective of nationality and location, cosmeticians, like dressmakers, adopted French names and titles to give that added je ne sais quoi to their business. In London you could visit Mme Day for all complexion disorders and Mme Elvira to get rid of that saggy chin and baggy neck. In New York you could attend Mme Hudson's School of beauty culture or 're-normalise the colloidal system of the body', and restore 'lithesome youth' with Ortosan 'an authentic scientific method created and perfected by Mme Louise Hernance under the guidance of eminent European physicians'.

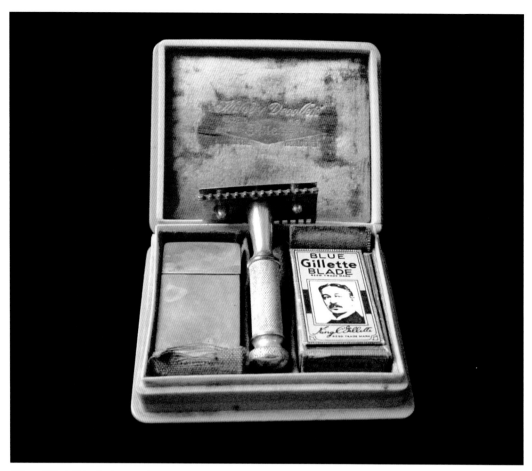

Gillette Milady Décolleté razor, 1916.

SELLING BEAUTY: Are you wrinkly? Are you hairy? Do you smell?

With so many new 'Madames' entering the market with their miracle creams and exotic foreign products more traditional companies had to rethink their marketing strategies. Pond's revitalised flagging demand with celebrity endorsement. In a hugely successful campaign beginning in 1924 the company published full page testimonials from three reigning queens, six princesses, and a bevy of European aristocrats and American society belles: Queen Marie of Romania 'one of the most beautiful and fascinating women of Europe', Lady Diana Manners 'the most beautiful complexion in the world', Mrs Reginald Vanderbilt 'Did you ever see such grace?' According to the oleaginous copy all these fashionable beauties owed their 'jasmine white, satin soft, and chiffon velvet' skin to the daily application of Pond's cold and vanishing creams. In fact, presaging the photo-shop perfection of Twenty-first Century advertisements, the photographic studio would spend up to a week retouching each negative.

Depilation

Another American company to benefit from the new preoccupation with the body beautiful was Gillette, founded in 1904 when travelling salesman King Camp Gillette patented the disposable safety razor – a brilliant invention in that it was a product that men used everyday and that could

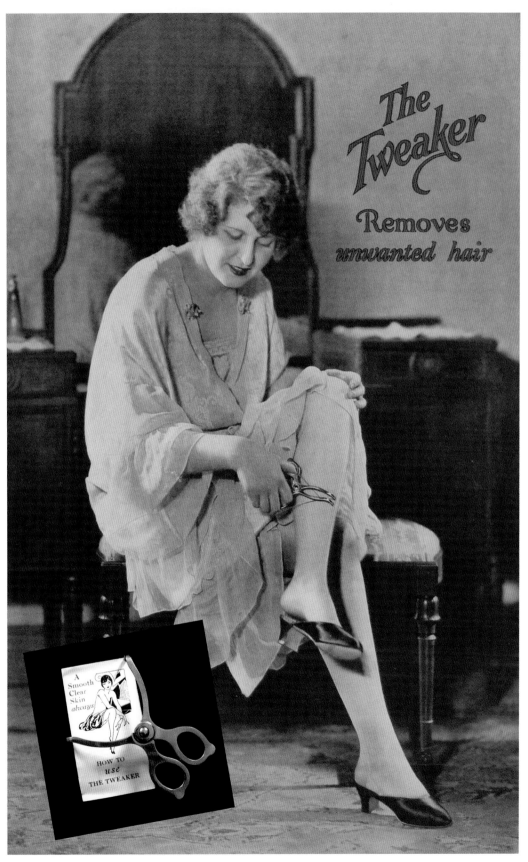

The Tweaker which 'Removes unwanted hair', 1920s.

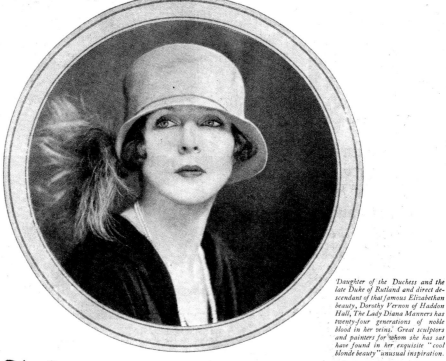

Daughter of the Duchess and the late Duke of Rutland and direct descendant of that famous Elizabethan beauty, Dorothy Vernon of Haddon Hall, The Lady Diana Manners has twenty-four generations of noble blood in her veins. Great sculptors and painters for whom she has sat have found in her exquisite "cool blonde beauty" unusual inspiration.

The Lady DIANA MANNERS

believes in this complete means of rejuvenating the skin

· · · *a deep refreshing cleansing*
· · · *a delicate finish and protection*

ARISTOCRAT by birth and breeding from the crown of her golden bobbed head to her slender silk-stockinged ankles, the Lady Diana Manners is a true democrat at heart. She adores beauty for its own pure sake, but also for the happiness it brings to the whole world. And she is genuinely interested in the happiness, and loveliness of other women.

This famous English beauty who knows the importance of keeping her own skin as white and delicate as hepaticas in May, and who does it by bathing it in a delicious cleansing cream, tells other women how they, too, can keep their clear-skinned freshness.

"Every woman," she says, "can have a fresh undimmed complexion if she'll take care of her skin, devoting a little time each day to keeping it supple and protected. I know that she can effectively accomplish this loveliness by using Pond's Two Creams."

Every night before retiring, and during the day, especially after exposure to the weather, cleanse your face and neck with Pond's Cold Cream, patting it lavishly over your skin. Let it stay on long enough for its pure oils to seep down into your pores and bring to the

surface the dust, dirt and powder which choke them. Wipe off all the cream and dirt and repeat, closing the pores with a dash of cold water or a rub with ice. If your skin is dry, after the nightly cleansing leave some of the cream on until morning.

After every cleansing with Pond's Cold Cream, except the bed-time one, finish and protect your skin with a delicate film of Pond's Vanishing Cream. It is a perfect base for holding your powder—holds it evenly, smoothly and long and causes it to blend ever so naturally with rouge. Pond's Vanishing Cream protects the skin, too, from hurtful soot, dust, wind and cold, keeping it fresh and supple for hours.

Pond's Cold Cream now comes in large jars! Both creams in smaller sizes of jars and in tubes.

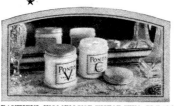

★

BEAUTIFUL WOMEN USE THESE TWO CREAMS

FREE OFFER—Mail this coupon for free tubes of these Two Creams and instructions for using them.

The Pond's Extract Company, Dept. M
135 Hudson Street, New York City

Please send me your free tubes of Pond's Two Creams.

Name. . . . .

Address. . . . .

City. . . . . .State. . . . . .

In using advertisements see page 6   95

Pond's Cream advertisement featuring Lady Diana Manners, 1925.

161

Friends ARE TOO TIMID TO TELL HER . . .
and she *permits*
a condition ABHORRENT to everyone

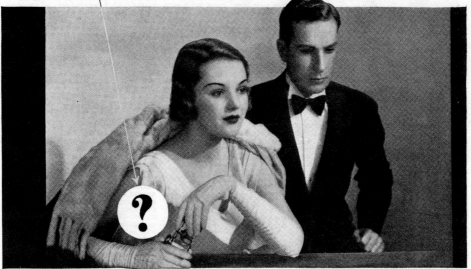

ENTRUST YOUR *Charm* TO NOTHING LESS SURE THAN ODO·RO·NO

You'd blush with humiliation . . . you'd be shamed to tears if you knew how needlessly you offend other people.

And you *do* offend them—you *do* lose friends—when you permit perspiration to go unchecked. For your own underarm odor . . . so unbearable to others . . . is seldom perceptible to you. Rarely do you know your own offense.

Your underarms may even *seem* dry, but perspiration moisture in the confined armpits quickly forms an acid that ruins dresses and turns friends against you. Even frequent bathing is never enough.

If you care at all what other people think, you'll insist on a deodorant that's trustworthy and sure. You *can* trust Odorono . . . a physician's formula . . . to protect you so completely that your mind is always free of all fear of offending.

ODO·RO·NO is Sure

And by checking, safely and completely, all underarm moisture, it saves your dresses from ruinous stains. Actually it saves its cost fifty times a year, and all year long it protects you from loss of respect, loss of friends and social defeat.

Determine to get Odorono today. For quick, convenient use choose Instant Odorono. Use it daily or every other day for complete, continuous protection. For longest protection or special need, choose Odorono Regular and use it faithfully twice a week. Both Odoronos have the original sanitary applicator. Both come in 35c and 60c sizes.

ODO·RO·NO
Never Fails You

● The Odorono original sanitary applicator is easier and more convenient to use. It holds just enough liquid at a time, and it is washable, too.

Millions of women . . . in 73 countries all over the world . . . trust their charm only to Odorono's safe and sure protection. Odorono is sure and certain.

It's approved by Good Housekeeping, and used by doctors and nurses everywhere. Let no one think you undainty . . . be faithful to Odorono.

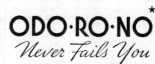
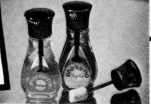

RUTH MILLER, THE ODORONO CO., Inc. Dept. 6-F4, 191 Hudson St., New York City (In Canada, address P.O. Box 2320, Montreal)
I enclose 10c for a special introductory bottle of Odorono with original sanitary applicator. (Check the type you wish to try) . . .
☐ Instant Odorono   ☐ Odorono Regular
Name
Address

EVERY product advertised is guaranteed—see page 6

Odorono advertisement, 1934.

LADIES' HOME JOURNAL September, 192

Even in those "trying days"

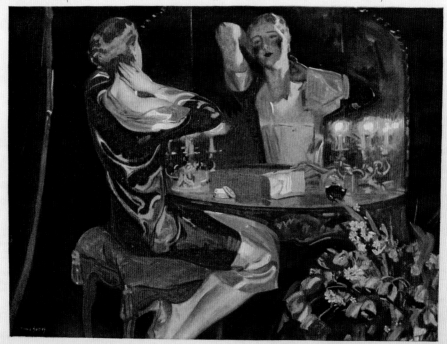

"Mum" preserves your daintiness

A confidential talk by
Winifred Sherman (Graduate Nurse)

A SHORT TIME AGO I wrote an advertisement in the Ladies' Home Journal, telling my readers that "Mum"—the famous perspiration deodorant—also assures absolute personal daintiness when used with the sanitary pad.

I want to further impress upon all who appreciate the importance of this subject that "Mum" not only is extremely effective in neutralizing all unpleasant odor, but also that it is gentle and soothing. Whether for the sanitary pad or for that other source of embarrassment—perspiration odor—"Mum" simply *deodorizes*, completely and lastingly. *It does nothing else.*

To the well-bred woman "Mum" is an essential part of the toilette. The use of "Mum" is her assurance that her feminine charm will be always above reproach.

In each jar of "Mum"—35c and 60c at your store —you will find an authoritative leaflet in which I have gone into the whole subject of daintiness very intimately. Or you may send for it with the coupon. You will be grateful for the information it contains, I feel sure.

"Mum" prevents all body odor

SPECIAL OFFER COUPON

Winifred Sherman, Mum Mfg. Co., Dept. J,
1106 Chestnut St., Philadelphia, Pa.

Enclosed is............for offer checked ☐ *Special Offer*—15c "Mum", for personal daintiness and 15c "Amoray" Talc, perfumed with rare and exotic fragrance—60c worth for 45c postpaid. ☐ Introductory size of "Mum" 10c postpaid. ☐ Send me free authoritative leaflet.

Name..

Address...

City...9-28

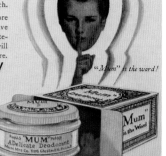

"Mum" is the word!

Mum deodorant advertisement, 1928.

be purchased over and over again. The only limitation to its multi-million sales potential was sex. Men shaved, women didn't or not at least until fashions began to change. With shorter skirts and sleeveless dresses, suddenly ankles and armpits were on display, providing new body areas for women to worry about and manufacturers to target.

In 1916 Gillette launched the Milady Décolleté, their first razor for women. Tiny and discreetly boxed lady shavers were soon to be found in every bathroom cabinet and the 1920s saw the flourishing of mass-produced cream and powder depilatories. 'Nothing is so repellent and disillusioning as hair growth on the arms of a woman,' warned a 1924 ad for 'Veet the new hair removal cream'. 'A New Freedom, a New Daintiness for Every Woman,' promised the Tweaker, though if you followed the instructions – using the contraption every day to tweak out unwanted hairs one by one – how much freedom you had was probably questionable.

Deodorising

It wasn't just hairy legs that women had to be concerned about. With the rise in sport and dancing came sweat, not a subject that ladies were used to hearing discussed. In 1919 OdoRoNo, an American deodorant for women, helped popularise the abbreviation BO for body odour. Their magazine advertising provided such a frank discussion of the moist and pungent unpleasantness that could lurk 'Within the Curve of a Woman's Arm' that 200 readers of *Ladies Home Journal* cancelled their subscriptions.

Sales of OdoRoNo however shot up by 112%. Manufacturers promised it would protect a lady 'from loss of friends, loss of respect and social defeat' and the deodorant came both in liquid form and powder, housed in an art deco style brass compact that could be slipped into a handbag. Perstik packaged their deodorant like a lipstick and 'Mum' cream deodorant came in a glass jar.

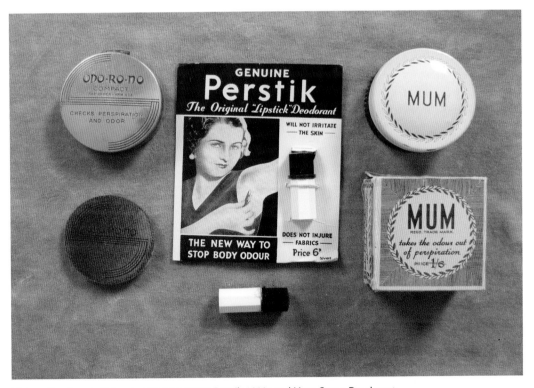

Vintage Deodorants: Odorono compact, 1930s, Perstik, 1930s, and Mum Cream Deodorant.

THEATRE MAGAZINE, MAY, 1926

This Ends Oily Skins

This remarkable new way of removing cleansing cream

Lightens darkish skins 4 or 5 shades—instantly
Holds make-up fresh for hours

Please accept a 7-day supply to try. See coupon below

HERE is a scientific discovery that will prove, no matter how long you have used cold cream, you have never removed it, and its accumulation of dirt, entirely from your skin . . . you have never removed it in gentle safety to your skin.

May we give you a 7-day supply, without charge, to try?

It is not a cloth, not a makeshift, *but an entirely new kind of material.* It contrasts the harshness of fibre or tissue methods with a softness that you'll love. It ends the "soiled towel" bother.

A scientific creation

We are makers of absorbents, are world authorities in this field.

On the urge of a noted dermatologist, we started out to perfect a thorough remover for cold cream . . . a right way that would remove it *all*, and *all* the pores' accumulations of dirt, grease and germ-laden residue with it.

Now that exactment has been met. We worked two years to do it. And we're told it marks one of the most important advancements in skin care known.

What it is

The name is KLEENEX—exquisitely dainty, inviting and immaculate—you use it, then discard it.

Scientifically aseptic, it reaches you white as snow, soft as down. It is 27 times as absorbent as an ordinary towel; 24 times as any fibre or tissue substitute.

Kleenex comes in two sizes — the Professional (sheets 9 by 10 inches) and the Boudoir size (sheets 6 by 7 inches) in exquisite flat handkerchief boxes to fit your dressing table drawer.

Today, largely on the advice of skin specialists, women are flocking to its use.

It will effect unique results in the texture and fineness of your skin; in the color and whiteness of your skin.

Combats oily skins and blemishes

You use cold cream to remove germ-laden accumulations. Old methods removed but part, rubbed the rest back in. That's where eruptions came . . . and those dark appearing skins.

* * *

It will correct oily skin and nose conditions amazingly. Oily skin indicates cold cream *left in* the skin. The pores exude it. That's why you must powder now so often

* * *

It will double and treble the effectiveness of your make-up . . . will make it last hours longer than before.

That's because it does what no other method can do, what no other even approximates; removes all dirt and grease from the pores.

Send the coupon

Please accept a 7-day supply free. Then see results yourself.

Just clip the coupon now before you forget. Mail it today for liberal supply at our expense. Prove these results for yourself.

At All Drug and Department Stores

Just make this test

Your make-up holds hours longer than before

Instead of towels, cloths, harsh fibre or paper makeshifts, you use this deliciously soft new material—27 times as absorbent!

First

*Remove every bit of germ-*laden matter, every particle of dirt, simply by wiping off face.

Then

—pay particular attention to the nose, so that it will be white and without shine.

Then

You discard the used sheets —no more soiling of towels.

KLEENEX
Sanitary Cold Cream Remover

Boudoir Size 35c
(Sheets 6 x 7 inches)

Professional Size 65c
(Sheets 9 x 10 inches)

7-Day Supply—FREE

KLEENEX CO.,   T-5
167 Quincy St., Chicago, Ill.

Please send without expense to me a sample packet of KLEENEX as offered.

Name...

Address...

Only one packet to a family.

1926 Kleenex Advertisement which claims, to 'end oily skin' and mysteriously to 'lighten darkish skin'.

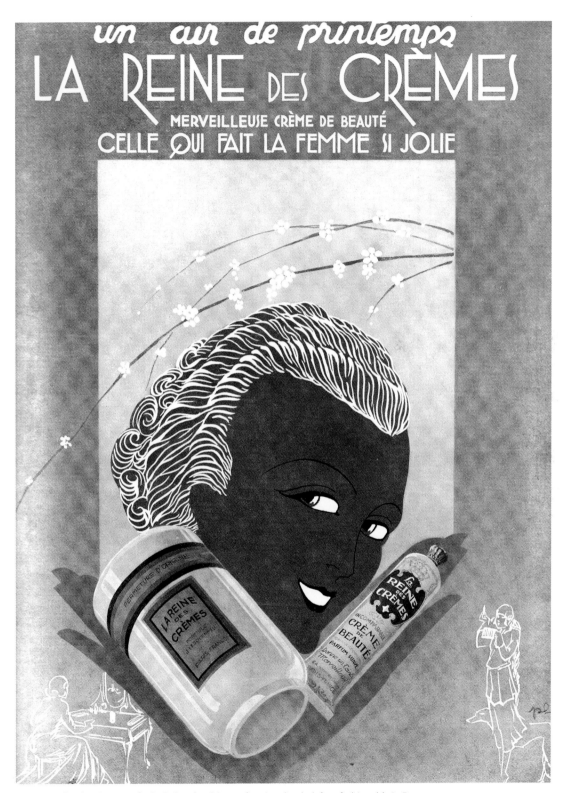

1931 French advertisement for La Reine des Crèmes showing the dark face fashionable in France.

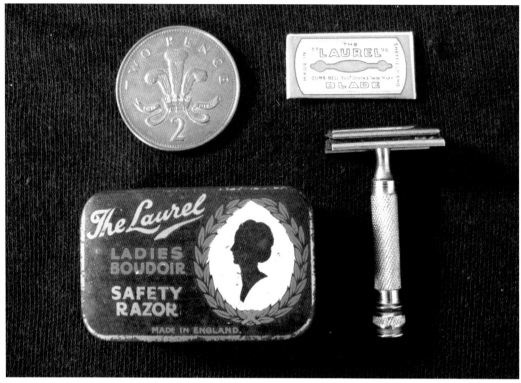

The Laurel Ladies Boudoir Safety Razor, 1930s. Shown next to a 2p coin to indicate its size, this tiny razor has a 2cm blade, making shaving the legs a lengthy process.

Ads in the 1920s recommended that 'the well-bred woman' should rub Mum both under her arms and onto her sanitary pads to ensure 'absolute personal daintiness' and avoid the 'embarrassment' of 'all unpleasant odor'.

Rather than just selling niceness and 'daintiness' (a favourite advertising word of the period), manufacturers of health and beauty products had discovered that playing on female insecurity could be hugely profitable. A telling example was Listerine, developed in the 1880s and used in the professional health care field as a general, all-purpose antiseptic. In the 1920s the manufacturers wanted to expand into the domestic market and when a company scientist mentioned the liquid could also be used to combat halitosis, they'd found their usp. A famous advertisement featured the 'pathetic' story of Edna, 'often a bridesmaid but never a bride', who was approaching her 'tragic' thirtieth birthday, still a spinster because of bad breath; 'a condition that you, yourself, rarely know when you have it. And even your closest friends won't tell you.' Suddenly everyone was worried about halitosis and Listerine sales went from $100,000 per year in 1921 over $4 million in 1927.

Personal Hygiene

In the 1920s a whole range of new beauty basics suddenly appeared on the market, typically pioneered in America. During WW1 US paper manufacturers Kimberley-Clark had developed a cellulose substitute for cotton that was used for gas mask filters and bandages. Cellu-cotton's first civilian appearance was as disposable feminine napkins, launched by the company in 1921 and far more convenient than traditional, washable rags. The success of Kotex (so-called for the cotton texture) helped inspire the creation of another famous brand.

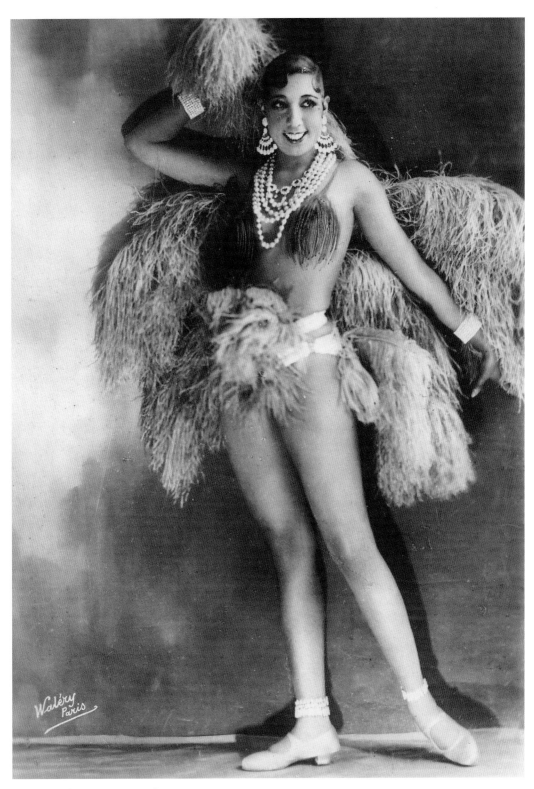

Josephine Baker vintage postcard, 1920s.

Kleenex was introduced to the US market in 1924 purely as a cold cream remover, the name reflecting its cleansing purpose as well as linking it to the Kimberley-Clark product range. To the firm's surprise however they received reports that people were blowing their noses on these luxury facial tissues. In 1926 they published two advertisements; one showing Kleenex being used as a cold cream remover and the other as a hygienic, throwaway handkerchief. The second inspired the largest customer response. The company changed their advertising to 'Don't Carry a Cold in Your Pocket' and the word Kleenex became synonymous for paper hankie. 'Baby Gays' were another disposable US innovation, created in 1923 by Polish-born American Leo Gerstenzang. The cotton swabs were devised for cleaning infants' ears but in 1926 when the manufacturers realized that adults were using them too – particularly for cosmetics – the name was changed to Q-tips (Q standing for Quality) and the swabs became a dressing table favourite as well as a nursery necessity.

For manufacturers the ladies' dressing table was an increasingly important target and looking (and smelling) good was big business. As Aldous Huxley reported in 1929 beauty was now the fourth largest industry in the USA – coming just behind automobiles, the movie industry and bootlegging. What with all the 'Soaps, skin foods, lotions, hair preservers and hair removers , powders, paints, pastes, pills that dissolve your fat from inside, bath salts that dissolve it from without, instruments for rubbing your fat away, foods that are guaranteed not to make you fat at all, machines that give you electric shocks, engines that massage and exercise your muscles … A face can cost as much in upkeep as a Rolls Royce.'

OOH LA LA! – Parisian Beauty

Yet while post-war women were enthusiastically encouraged to deodorise, moisturise and to keep slim, up until the first half of the 1920s, very overt use of cosmetics was regarded by many with some suspicion, and dismissed as either 'fast' or 'French' which amounted much to the same thing. Although they eulogised Parisian couture, magazines were often critical about continental maquillage. 'Parisiennes began to look like a race of quadroons,' sneered English *Vogue* in 1923 reporting on the recent winter fashion for brown face make-up.

Thanks to fewer clothes, more outdoor sports, and Coco Chanel (who allegedly acquired a tan by accident whilst holidaying in the South of France on her lover, the Duke of Westminster's, yacht) a brown skin became fashionable for the first time and not just on the Riviera.

Dancer Josephine Baker, 'the Black Pearl', 'the Panther with the golden claws', left America for Paris to star in La Revue Negre in 1925. Appearing at the Théâtre des Champs Elysées, then at the Folies Bergère, Baker charlestoned onto the stage wearing virtually nothing but a string of sixteen bananas round her waist, some sparkly jewellery and expertly applied make-up: grease to make her cropped hair shiny smooth, black lipstick to emphasise her large laughing mouth, kohl to outline her rolling, humorous eyes, and a specially blended powder to set off that 'magnificent dark body'. Baker showed the French that black was beautiful and took Paris by storm. Admirers showered her with expensive gifts and she received a reported 1,500 marriage proposals. Men wanted to sleep with her and women wanted to look like her – slicking down their hair with 'Bakerfix' brillantine and darkening their skin with tinted powder and cream to look like 'the black Venus'.

Not everyone however was quite so enthusiastic. 'Vulgar,' sneered Mistinguett, reigning queen of the French music hall, who dubbed this new American rival 'Banana tits'.

The highest paid performer of the day, Mistinguett was famous for her beautiful legs (insured in 1919 for 500,000F), her towering plumed headdresses and ostrich feather trains (pioneering what was to become the standard showgirl costume from Paris to Las Vegas), her legion of lovers (including the young Maurice Chevalier), her vile temper, and her opulent make-up; decorating her body with luminous paint and her eyes with brilliant colours.

Some of the most enthusiastic promoters of make-up in 1920s Paris were women who took their clothes off for a living: music hall performers, models, and demimondaines.

Kiki de Montparnasse (1901-1953) enjoyed all these professions. Actress, painter, artist's model and good-time girl, Kiki sat for some of the most progressive artists of the decade, including her lover Man Ray who immortalised her in his photograph *Le Violon d'Ingres*. Everyone who

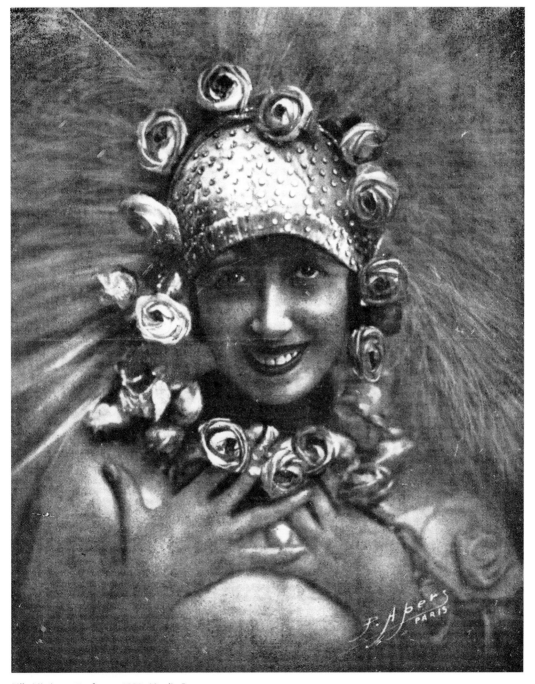

Mlle Mistinguett – from a 1920s Moulin Rouge programme

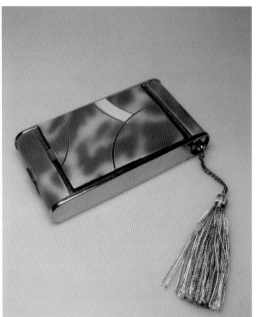

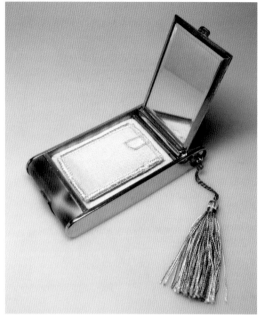

Above and Below Left: 1930s Camera-style compact closed and open showing cigarettes and a powder well. *Gray's Antiques Market.* **Below Right:** Modern compact showing 1930 poster of Josephine Baker: Casino de Paris by Zig. *Louis Gaudin*

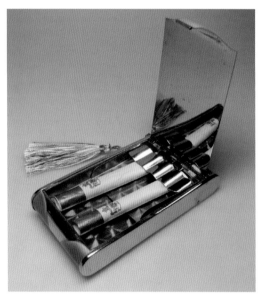

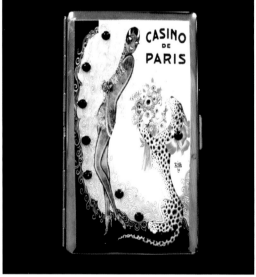

met Kiki remarked on her sexiness and her make-up. 'Her maquillage was a work of art in itself … her mouth painted a deep scarlet that emphasised the sly erotic humor of its contours. Her face was beautiful from every angle,' wrote the Canadian poet John Glassco in his *Memoirs of Montparnasse.* In her own autobiography written at the age of only twenty-eight, Kiki recalled how she distracted herself from a poor and wretched upbringing by decoration – reddening her cheeks with geranium petals and getting sacked from a bakery because she darkened her

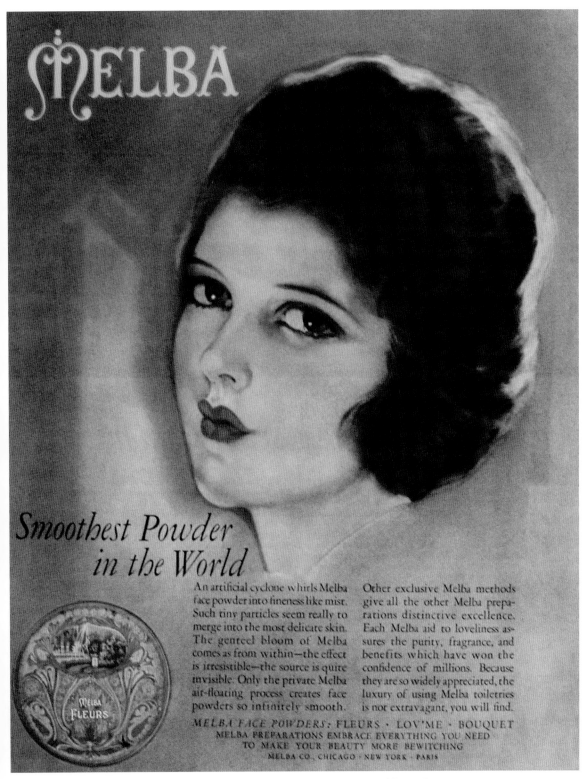

MELBA

Smoothest Powder in the World

An artificial cyclone whirls Melba face powder into fineness like mist. Such tiny particles seem really to merge into the most delicate skin. The genteel bloom of Melba comes as from within—the effect is irresistible—the source is quite invisible. Only the private Melba air-floating process creates face powders so infinitely smooth.

Other exclusive Melba methods give all the other Melba preparations distinctive excellence. Each Melba aid to loveliness assures the purity, fragrance, and benefits which have won the confidence of millions. Because they are so widely appreciated, the luxury of using Melba toiletries is not extravagant, you will find.

MELBA FACE POWDERS: FLEURS · LOV'ME · BOUQUET
MELBA PREPARATIONS EMBRACE EVERYTHING YOU NEED
TO MAKE YOUR BEAUTY MORE BEWITCHING
MELBA CO., CHICAGO · NEW YORK · PARIS

1926 Advertisement for Melba powder, showing a typical flapper face.

eyebrows with burnt matchsticks. When she went out in the evenings she painted her toenails and rouged her knees, and friends recalled that she was never seen without her handbag, inside which was a range of paints in vivid artificial colours, which she used to make her eyes match her dress or her earrings.

Kiki happily admitted to selling her body when she needed money, and that very same make-up filled handbag landed her in prison when she used it to hit a policeman.

MAKE-UP – STILL NAUGHTY AND NOT QUITE NICE

With such bohemian characters pioneering colourful cosmetics, small wonder that in more establishment circles face-painting still wasn't considered quite the done thing.

Vogue might have declared in 1919 that 'No one thinks of leaving the house nowadays without powder and lipstick, purse, notebook and smoking paraphernalia to which the latest addition is the gold briquette for lighting the perpetual cigarette,' yet the bright young things who sported these accessories came in for a good deal of criticism. *Vogue* itself admitted that there was nothing remotely appealing about 'a siren with a "stinker" between her lips' and girls who experimented with make-up were likely to have their face scrubbed by outraged parents. Writing in 1919 the young debutante Barbara Cartland described her chalk white powdered face and bright red lips 'subject of much criticism and many arguments'.

'The decadent and degenerate poisons of Paris infect our fashions,' thundered the *Daily Express* in 1920 disgusted by this 'absolutely brazen display' of body-hugging clothes and painted faces. 'The remedy is the lash of public opinion. It ought to be applied without delay.'

Fashion magazines of the early twenties carried very few advertisements for cosmetics and successful manufacturers of beauty products actively sought to distance themselves from face painting. 'The lovely women who follow Elizabeth Arden's method are never dependent upon artifice to create an effect of beauty,' boasted Elizabeth Arden smugly in 1924. That same year Helena Rubinstein promised that her creams would create a truly individual beauty: 'Not the mere application of "camouflage cosmetics" to cover up skin defects and reduce every woman's face to doll-like, uninteresting sameness.' Although Coco Chanel was responsible for popularising suntanning and for creating Chanel No.5 in 1921 – the first perfume to bear the name of a designer and arguably the most famous scent of all time – she too was unenthusiastic about extravagant make-up, blaming its use on the gay influence she felt was corrupting the simplicity of women's fashion that she had fought so hard to achieve.

'Homosexuals … They are the ones who inspire hats no women can wear, the ones who acclaim unwearable dresses … They are the only men who love make-up and red nail polish.'

But patently they weren't. In the USA in particular, pancake make-up, twist-up lipsticks, scarlet nail varnish, and extravagantly made up movie stars, were all being pioneered and promoted by a generation of red-blooded males – cosmetics manufacturers, Hollywood moguls, hard bitten businessmen – who while making a fortune from the beauty business would help change the way women thought about their faces and bodies for ever.

CHAPTER FIVE

Hooray for Hollywood
Beauty in the 1930s

HOLLYWOOD HAD a huge influence on the development and popularisation of cosmetics. With the launch of the motion picture industry in the early 1900s, performer's faces were magnified to unprecedented levels, were seen by more people than ever before, and had the potential to become world-famous. Initially film companies tried to keep their actors anonymous (worried that they would want more money), but the public demanded to know their identities and flocked to movies featuring their favourite performers.

This audience interest led to the foundation of the studio star system, in which the great film companies masterminded the actor's persona, both on and off the silver screen. The studio publicity departments invented new personal histories for their stars, and where necessary changed their names: Marion Morrison became John Wayne, Lucille Le Sueur (which sounded too much like sewer) Joan Crawford. The studio's make-up and hairdressing artists changed their looks. They created instantly recognisable features; Jean Harlow's platinum blonde hair, Joan Crawford's post box lips, Marlene Dietrich's elevated eyebrows. They concealed physical imperfections: Dietrich's nose was made to look straighter on film by drawing a silver line down the middle; Garbo's crooked teeth were fixed and her white blonde lashes darkened with mascara; Rita Hayworth had her brow line painfully raised with electrolysis; John Wayne opted simply for a toupee. Hair and make-up were hugely important in realising the Hollywood dream, the 'rags to riches' fairy tale of the ordinary person – from a small town or the wrong side of the tracks – who could be transformed into a star.

Cosmetics were also crucial to the medium of cinema itself. Close ups and strong lighting necessitated a new make-up. Traditional stick greasepaint was too heavy, coating the face under a thick, unnatural layer that cracked in the heat. The first cinema foundation was invented by Max Factor, 'the father of modern cosmetics' and the man who popularised the word 'make-up', transforming it from a theatrical term into something found in every woman's handbag.

MAX FACTOR (c.1872–1938)
Born in Lodz, Poland, Max Faktor rose from humble Jewish origins to become wigmaker and cosmetic artist to the Imperial Russian Grand Opera; before emigrating to the USA where he changed the spelling of his name to Max Factor and set up a theatrical make-up shop in Los Angeles in 1909. He was the right man in the right place at the right time. In 1910, D.W. Griffith

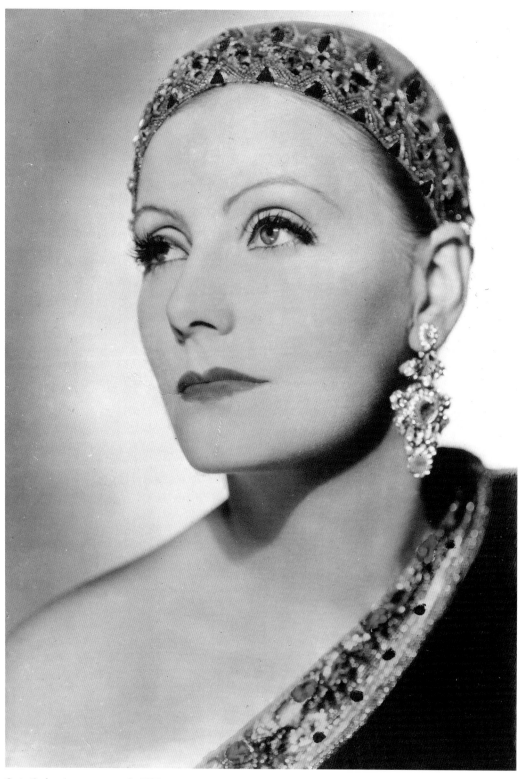

Greta Garbo vintage postcard c.1930.

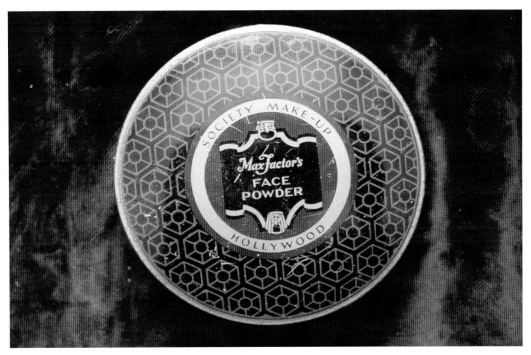

Max Factor Society Make-up Face Powder, 1930s

made the first film ever shot in Hollywood. Attracted by fine weather, good locations and cheap land, the new generation of moviemakers flooded to California. By 1911 over 150 companies were based in the Los Angeles area and by 1914 Hollywood had become the film capital of the world. That same year Max Factor released the first make-up devised specifically for the movies – a flexible greasepaint that came in cream form, that moved (without cracking) with the actors' faces, and that was eventually supplied in a hygienic, convenient tube. This innovation was followed by a host of others that were to literally change the face of the cinema.

In 1914, Factor persuaded Cecil B. DeMille to rent real hair wigs for *The Squaw Man*, far more natural looking than cheap artificial substitutes – but so expensive that Factor insisted his sons should play extras in this and subsequent Westerns so that they could keep an eye on the valuable native American plaits during massacre scenes.

'Color Harmony' cosmetics, blended to suit individual complexions, were launched in 1918, much to the relief of the olive-skinned Rudolf Valentino, who was sick of the deathly pallor created by traditional foundation. Max Factor also pioneered lipgloss, the lip brush and waterproof make-up (contributing to the success of swimming star Esther Williams).

With the arrival of Technicolor, make-up devised for black and white movies became unintentionally colourful too. Faces that looked perfect in the studio appeared red, green and blue on film as they picked up reflections from surrounding objects. In 1928, Max Factor developed a new 'Panchromatic' make-up devised for colour film, then in 1937 he launched Pan-Cake, a solid cake of foundation, applied with a sponge which provided a smooth, non reflective, matt finish. 'Never before in a colour motion picture have the players looked so natural and realistic,' enthused one movie critic. Pan-Cake became the industry staple, then when it was retailed commercially at the end of the thirties, a public favourite, claiming to be the fastest and largest selling single item in the history of cosmetics.

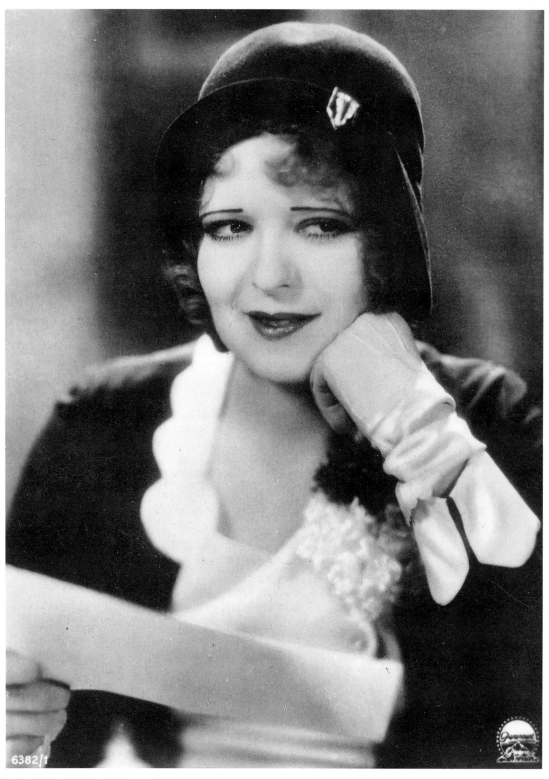

6382/1

Clara Bow vintage postcard c.1920s.

VAMPS & IT GIRLS

New cosmetics not only made individual stars look their best but created a new series of archetypes for women to emulate.

In *A Fool There Was* (1915) Theda Bara pioneered the image of the vamp – short for vampire – a glamorous, heartless seductress, instantly recognisable by her exotic (usually Eastern) appearance, dark hair and extravagant make-up emphasising eyes and lips. Studio publicists claimed Theda Bara was the daughter of an Arabian princess and a French artist, that she was raised on serpent's blood, and that her name was an anagram of Arab Death. In reality Theodosia (Theda) Goodman was a Jewish girl born in Cincinnati and Bara was a contraction of Baranger, her grandfather's name.

The vamps, Theda Bara, Pola Negri, and Nita Naldi portrayed foreign femme fatales with heavily kohled eyes and outrageous costumes (snakes and tiger skins were favourite accessories). A more accessible look was provided by another silent movie archetype: the It Girl.

Released in 1927, the *It Girl*, the story of a shop assistant who falls in love with the owner of the department store, was based on a novella by British author and Hollywood Grande Dame Elinor Glyn. 'It,' she explained in her famously sonorous voice, 'is the peculiar fascination that makes someone immensely attractive to all men and all women. 'It' is animal magnetism … 'It' is always utterly unselfconscious … 'It' is one of the rarest gifts in the world …'. In other words, 'It' was sex appeal and the woman who had 'It' in spades was the film's star Clara Bow.

A Brooklyn babe – gum chewing, wise-cracking, flirtatious – Bow shimmied her way out of an abusive, poverty stricken childhood, by winning a beauty contest, which led to a screen test and a film career in which playing manicurists, shop assistants and waitresses, she came to epitomise the modern American girl – the liberated flapper.

Clara Bow became an icon for thousands of young women who bought 50c copies of the Clara Bow cloche hat from *Sears Catalog* and followed her every move. Clara was famous for her red hair, which she set off by driving round Los Angeles in a red Packard roadster filled with her red chow dogs. When fans found out that she used henna, sales of the hair dye tripled. Women plucked their eyebrows and kohled their eyes to imitate her wide-eyed ingénue look and applying red lipstick in a heart shape was known as the Clara Bow.

LIPSTICK LOVELIES

Movie stars (and their make-up artists) did much to popularise the use of lipstick. Ziegfield Follies dancer turned silent movie actress Mae Murray became known as 'the girl with the bee stung lips', a style created by Max Factor to resolve a technical problem. Under studio lights, lip pomade melted and ran over the star's face. Factor prevented this by ignoring Mae's natural lip line, covering her mouth with a base of greasepaint, then applying two thumb prints of coloured pomade to the upper lips and one thumb print to the lower lip, which he then outlined with a lip brush, creating a rosebud pout that became one of the classic looks of the period, sported by stars ranging from Bebe Daniels to the first cartoon flapper Betty Boop.

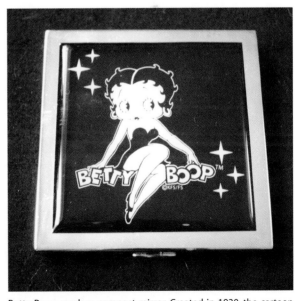

Betty Boop modern compact mirror. Created in 1930, the cartoon flapper remains a popular icon.

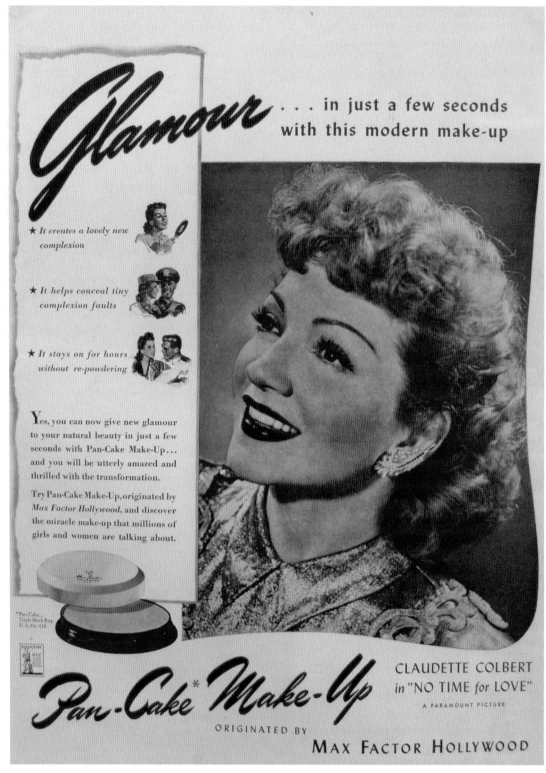

Max Factor Pan-Cake Make-up advertisement, starring Claudette Colbert, early 1940s.

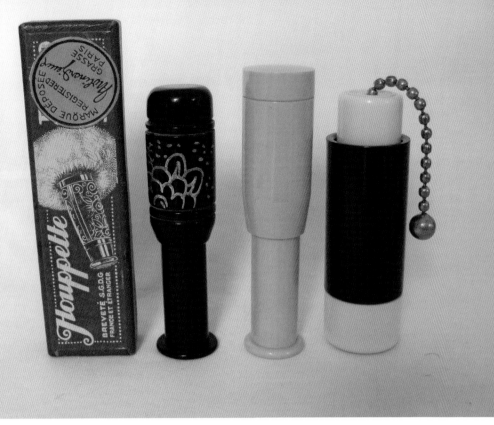

1930s portable powder puffs, the Houppette shown (in two colours) and the Lamkin. When closed and capped they could be safely carried in a handbag.

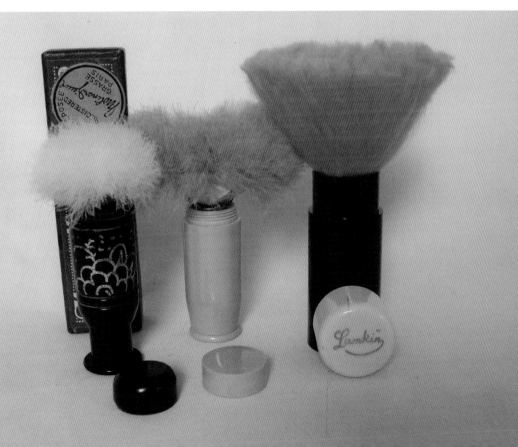

In the early thirties Joan Crawford wanted to distinguish herself from this posse of 'It girls' and juveniles, and went to Max Factor for a new image. Again ignoring the natural lip line, Max Factor ran a thick layer of colour over and beyond her lips, giving her the full and sensual shape which he called 'The Smear' but which was sold to her legions of fans as 'hunter's bow lips'. Crawford's lips became her trademark, crucial to her predatory sexual appeal. 'She's slept with every male star at MGM except Lassie,' commented her famous rival Bette Davis. Not to be outdone, Bette Davis had a mouth makeover from Ern Westmore, member of a famous family of Hollywood cosmetic artists whose House of Westmore Beauty Salon on Sunset Boulevard was a favourite venue for movie stars. Ern Westmore lipstick-ed over the Cupid's bow to give Davis her signature 'slash' mouth. Large eyes were her other defining feature. 'When I die, they'll probably auction off my false eyelashes,' claimed Davis, who as well as false eyelashes, favoured lashings of brown mascara. 'Miss Davis was always partial to covering up her face in motion pictures. She called it 'Art'. Others might call it camouflage – a cover-up for the absence of any real beauty,' sneered Joan Crawford, getting her own back.

But reality, beautiful or otherwise had very little to do with the appeal of Hollywood stars. The point of glamorous make-up was that it made you look and feel better. What women saw in the movies they wanted for themselves. By 1928 Max Factor's 'Society Make Up' (his retail line) was being distributed across the US; promoted by the stars for whom it had originally been created. 'Jean Harlow's beauty is always fascinating – Would You like to share her MAKE-UP SECRET?' enticed a typical Max Factor advertisement. The answer was of course yes. From being the preserve of actresses, show girls and ladies of the night, make-up had mutated into a daily necessity for women across the world and a huge market for its manufacturers.

MAKE-UP FOR THE MASSES

'Not so long ago the woman who used powder, to say nothing of rouge or lipstick, was literally as well as figuratively, beyond the pale. Today the situation has changed, but there has arisen instead the sin of not using make-up wisely and well,' warned *Vogue* in 1930. The question was no longer whether to wear make-up at all, but what to choose from an ever expanding range of products. Having virtually ignored cosmetics in the early twenties, by the 1930s women's magazines were featuring dedicated beauty columns providing tips and advice, whilst salons were offering an endless variety of services.

'The fastidious likes the very best in those dainty finishing touches such as powder, rouge and lipstick,' insisted Helena Rubinstein, who like Elizabeth Arden had conveniently forgotten her previous disdain for duplicitous 'camouflage cosmetics'. At

Max Factor ad starring Jean Harlow, 1934, the face of the moment.

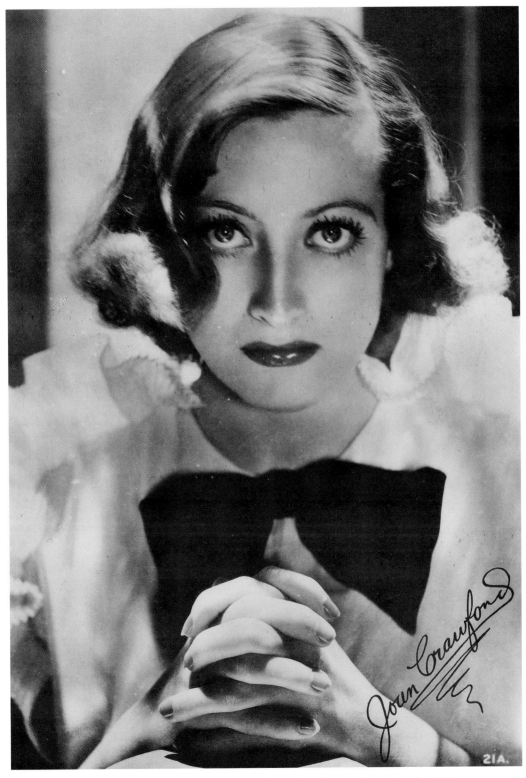

Vintage postcard of Joan Crawford whose heavily made-up lips and eyes became her trademark, c. 1930.

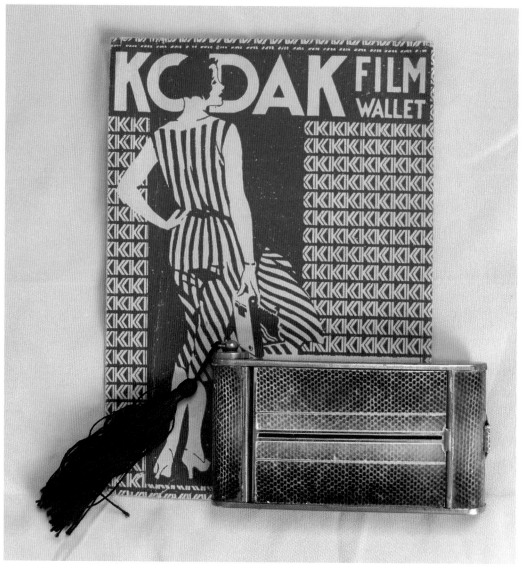

Kodak film wallet with camera shaped compact – 1930s.

Rubinstein's salons you could now not only purchase 'exciting rouges', 'thrilling lipsticks' and 'enticing eye make-up', but she was also offering classes in 'the art of "making up" effectively and correctly', and makeovers for special occasions. 'The Season's on! You are being presented perhaps? Going to Ascot –certainly! And being photographed constantly … State Occasions demand special make-up, have it done by experts. It only takes half an hour and only costs 12/6.'

The rise of photography and the instant snap, as opposed to the carefully prepared studio portrait, certainly caused women to be more aware of how they looked and increased the need to 'put a face on'. 'Most of us have sustained the horror that comes from recognising some beady-eyed bag in the current illustrated papers as a portrait of ourselves at this or that hunt ball,' moaned *Vogue* in 1934. 'What,' *Vogue* asked Miss Mayle of Cyclax, 'can people do to prevent themselves looking like frights in hunt ball snap shots?'

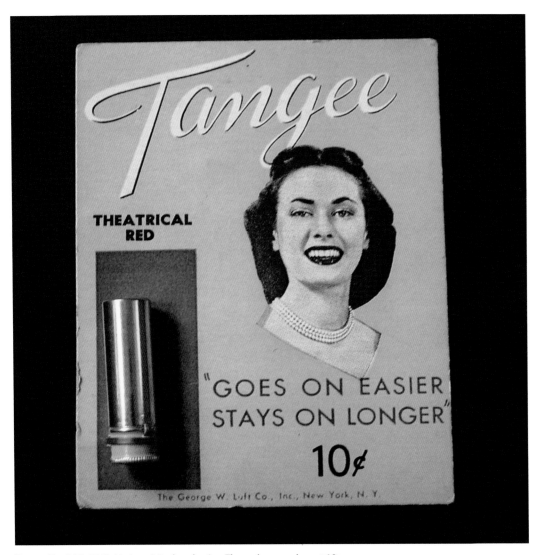

Tangee lipstick(c.1940s) in its original packaging. The make-up only cost 10c.

A popular thirties vanity case was inspired by the flat cameras of the period – the compact opened with a simulated shutter button; held rouge and powder in one side; cigarettes in the other; whilst the 'film winder' pulled out to reveal a lipstick. In 1928 Eastman Kodak got together with cosmetics firm Richard Hudnut to produce the Vanity Kodak Ensemble, a mirrored leather carrying case housing a real Kodak camera and a tango compact containing rouge, powder and lipstick; so that a lady could always look her best.

It wasn't just the wealthy who were becoming more aware of make-up and their photographic image. Woolworth's highly successful marketing strategy was that nothing in their high street stores cost over sixpence (2.5p). One of the shop's most popular single products during the 1930s was the Woolworth '6d' camera, and among their best-selling general lines were cosmetics: Tangee lipstick, Cutex nail polish, novelty powder puffs, compacts, manicure sets. Instant beauty, easily available at a price that pretty much everybody could afford and that attracted some unexpected customers.

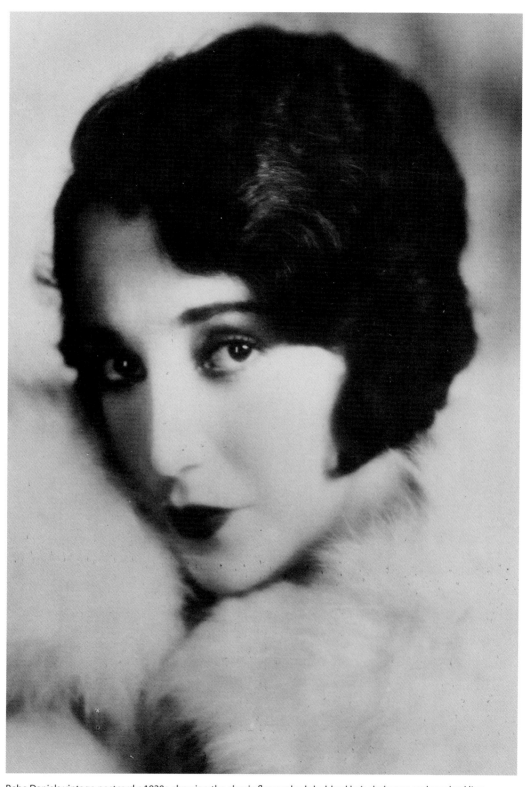

Bebe Daniels vintage postcard c.1920s, showing the classic flapper look: bobbed hair, dark eyes and rosebud lips.

British newspapers of the 1920s and 1930s worried about the increasing proliferation of 'painted boys' trolling the city streets. As historian Matt Houlbrook reports in *The Man with the Powder Puff in Interwar London*, being caught with a lipstick or compact in a trouser pocket was itself almost enough to get a man arrested for male importuning; and cosmetics and powder puffs featured as evidence in a number of period homosexual prosecutions. The fact that men could actually buy these items reflects the increasing availability of make-up, which had moved out of the exclusive beauty salon and the upper class department store and on to the ordinary high street. Boots opened their 1000th store in 1933 and two years later launched their famous No7 beauty brand, advertised as 'The Modern Way to Loveliness'.

In America too make-up was being produced for every level of the market. In 1916 Charles Jundt took over the hairdressing salon of the Ritz-Carlton hotel in New York, and in 1926 he launched the highly exclusive cosmetics line 'Charles of the Ritz', which supplied hand-blended powders to suit a lady's individual complexion. At the same time make-up had become a staple of the five and dime stores, and even during the Depression cosmetic sales continued to rise. A 10c lipstick provided a quick and cheap pick-me-up and wasn't just a frivolity. Trying to keep well groomed under duress was not only a way of preserving your self-esteem but could even help you find a job. 'Look your best,' advised the beauty columnists, 'and you will do your best.'

In the few years since World War I there had been a dramatic revolution. Far from suggesting loose morals or rebellious youth, make-up (carefully applied of course as magazines never ceased to remind their readers) had become a symbol of respectability; the mark of a woman who cared for herself and for others, and who loved her husband enough not to 'let herself go'. In Britain cosmetics were available everywhere, from local chemists to exclusive Mayfair beauty salons. Across the Atlantic, according to a 1930s advertising agency report, American women were using 375,000,000 boxes of face powder, 240,000,000 cakes of dry rouge and three thousand miles of lipstick each year. Cosmetics had become a multi-million dollar industry and the only thing that could halt the expansion of the beauty business across the globe was a world war.

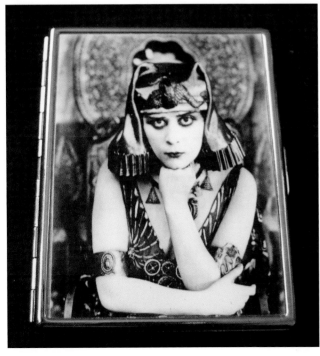

Modern compact decorated with a vintage picture of Theda Bara in vamp makeup.

CHAPTER SIX

On the Art Deco Dressing Table

Make-up Comes of Age

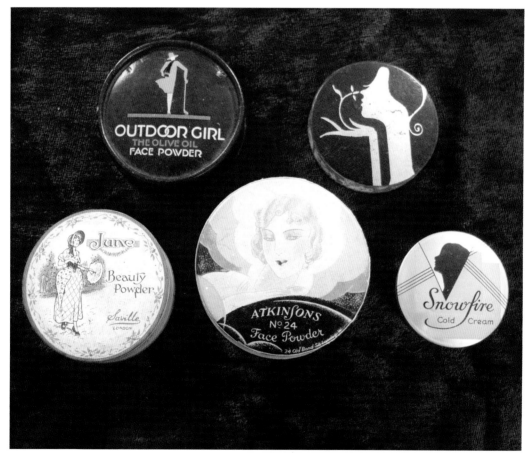

A collection of period powder boxes: Outdoor Girl; Tokalon; June by Saville: Atkinson's No.24; and a Snowfire cold cream tin, 1920s/30s.

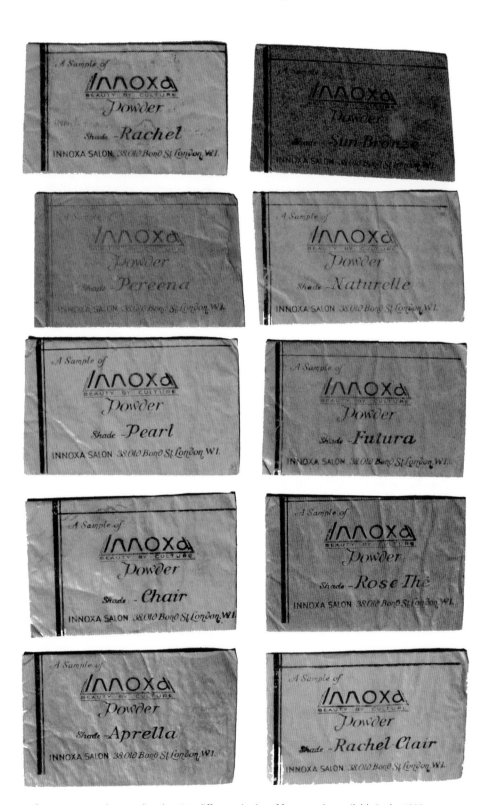

Collection of 10 Innoxa powder samples, showing different shades of face powder available in the 1930s.

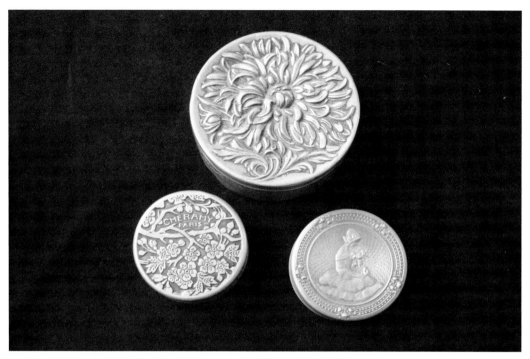

Aluminium powder boxes c.1920s – Cheramy, Paris; Rimmel (flower top); Poudre Du Barry (kneeling girl).

THEIR MOTHERS might have been satisfied with a smear of cold cream and a dusting of powder, but the women of the 1920s and 30s had a far greater choice of products. The beauty business boomed; dressing tables became increasingly laden with new cosmetics and from mascara to the twist-up lipstick, much of the make-up we take for granted today was popularised between the two World Wars.

FACE MAKE-UP
By the 1920s powder and rouge were dressing table staples. 'It has become very nearly imperative for every well groomed woman to understand the right use, not only of powder but of rouge as well,' observed *Vogue* in 1921; but while no longer condemning these products beauty advisors had no hesitation in criticising those who didn't use them properly. 'Cosmetic powders are not supposed to act in the guise of plaster-of-Paris masks, to completely hide the features,' warned Florence Courtenay in *Physical Beauty* 1922. 'When it comes to using face powder remember that moderation means charm.'

Immediately after the First World War this was easier said than done because, as Barbara Cartland remembered, there was still comparatively little powder to choose from. 'There were only three shades obtainable, dead white, yellow and almost brown.'

The 1920s however saw a powder-puff explosion and by the end of the decade Coty was advertising ten true shades of powder – including ochre, rose, Rachel, natural, mauve, and Coty-tan. World War I had been the making of the French company. American soldiers returned home from Europe with Parisian perfumes and powders for their wives, and the name of Coty spread across the USA. Coty Inc. was established in Manhattan in 1922 and, when the company decided to go for the mass market selling their famous air-spun powder in smaller cardboard boxes, and slashing prices from $2.50 to $1, Coty became a brand leader with a multi-million turnover. Helena Rubinstein and Elizabeth Arden supplied a wide range of powders: other leading names (among many) included Lablache, Jonteel, Ponds, Innoxa and Mello-Glo, 'The face powder preferred by 2M of America's most beautiful women … perspiration from dancing and exercise does not affect it'. As well as being produced in different shades, scented powders came smelling of all the favourite perfumes of the day ranging from Richard Hudnut's Three Flowers to Bourjois' Evening in Paris. Beautifully decorated tins and cardboard powder boxes provided the perfect complement to art deco dressing tables, and with so many manufacturers competing in the market place, advertising and packaging became increasingly important.

The rouge pot was another cosmetic essential, although here again, warned the unrelenting Miss Florence Courtenay, care had to be taken. 'Most people use rouge paste badly – and while using rouge is no crime, using it badly is. What is more ridiculous than to see a woman flush through her rouge, and present on one and the same cheek two distinct shades of color, real and artificial.'

The harsh rouges and hectic tints of the early 1920s became increasingly sophisticated. Rouge came in various forms: liquid, cream, powder, rouge papers and in an expanding range of colours; rose pink, raspberry red, coral, carmine, tangerine. Tangee produced tins of cream rouge to tone with their lipstick. Helena Rubinstein's Red Geranium rouge and lipstick in 1925 promised 'a vivid, live, palpitating healthglow colouring'.

The 1930s saw the increasing influence of film make-up and the use of new foundation products such as Robert Douglas Hollywood Foundation Cream and most famously Max Factor's Pan-Cake, which was promoted by a bevy of flawlessly complexioned Hollywood stars in the late thirties and forties.

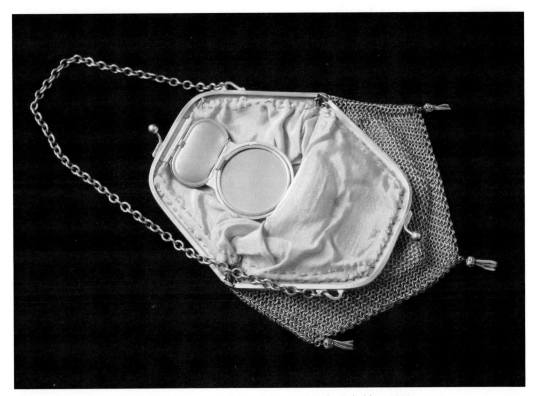

Solid silver mesh bag, made in Germany with integral vanity compact and coin holder c.1920s.

THE POWDER COMPACT

In the interwar years the powder compact was transformed from a guilty secret into a handbag necessity and something to show off.

Cosmetic companies recognised the advantages of this new publicity and sold powders and rouge in attractive portable containers. Coty's famous powder puff design – attributed to René Lalique and trademarked in 1914 – was used on slimline, metal compacts as well as full size powder boxes. The French firm Tokalon produced a rouge compact decorated with an art deco Pierrot; Houbigant (est.1775), France's oldest surviving perfumer; identified their cosmetic containers with a rococo style basket of flowers. Like Parisian couture, French cosmetics were the height of fashion, but British companies fought back. Yardley's famous lavender seller symbol (adapted in

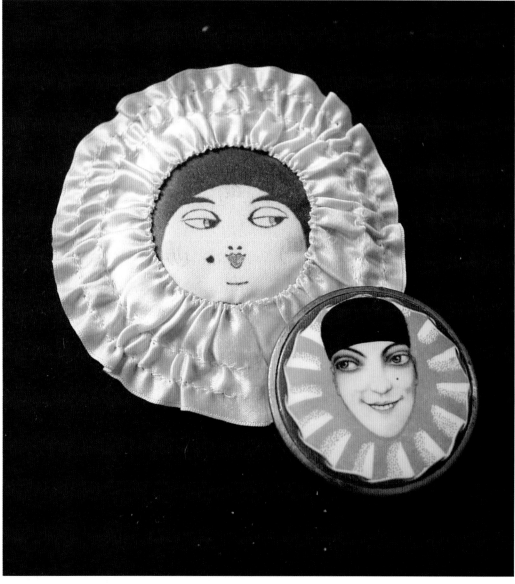

Tokalon rouge compact and a Pierrot powder puff, 1920s/30s.

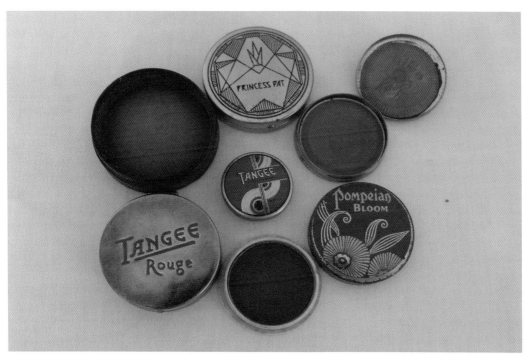

A collection of rouges open and closed, including Tangee, Princess Pat and Pompeian Bloom, dating from the 1920s/30s.

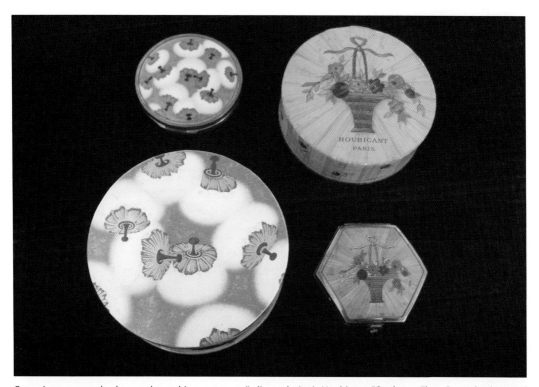

Coty air-spun powder box and matching compact (Lalique design); Houbigant "Quelques Fleurs" powder box and matching compact.

1913 from the *Cries of London* – an Eighteenth Century engraving by Francis Wheatley) appeared on compacts and skin care products, and when the spirit duty on lavender was removed in 1932, the company's turnover doubled.

As well as buying branded products, ladies decanted their make-up into personal compacts which came in every size, shape and material. 1920s compacts were often small (around 5cms in diameter). The 1930s saw the fashion for large circular flapjack compacts (so called after the flapjack pancake), measuring up to 10cms across and reflecting the influence of Hollywood (film stars were often portrayed at the dressing table) and the increasing size and strength of ladies' handbags, as the leather clutch took over from the delicate beaded pouch.

As make-up became increasingly acceptable, so compacts held more of it. Double or triple vanities, enamelled with stylish art deco patterns, came with compartments for rouge, powder, cigarettes and a pull-out lipstick. Tiny gilded boxes opened up to reveal a complete face-full of make-up. Plain compacts were designed for daytime use; elegant party cases coordinated with evening dress and reflected the latest flapper fashions. In the late 1920s, US firms such as Elgin American and Evans were producing delicate chained silver vanity cases, designed to dangle from a wrist or finger ring. The tango compact had a separate lipstick attached to its chain handle.

Manufacturers competed in design and decoration, patenting new mechanisms for grinding, sifting and dispensing powder, and devising ingenious cosmetic novelties. Compacts were hidden inside tiny teddy bears; a hairbrush came with a pull-out lipstick handle; a pocket fan concealed a vanity mirror. Miniature compacts could be worn as lockets or brooches and various patents were taken out for bracelets, with cunningly concealed vanity compartments.

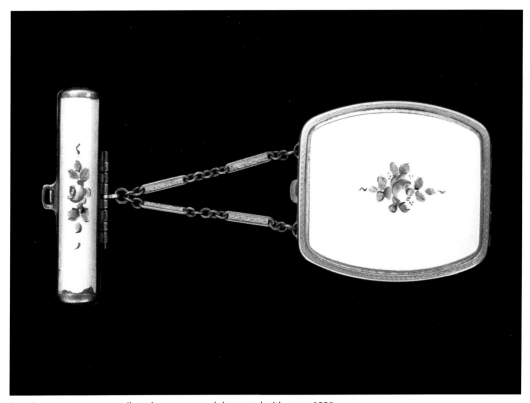

American tango compact, gilt and cream enamel decorated with roses, 1920s.

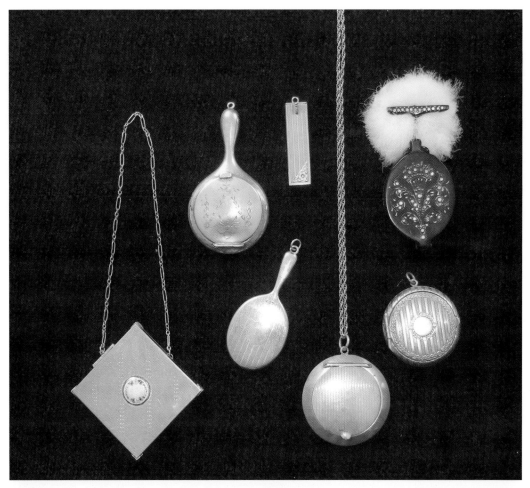

Compacts and vanity items from the 1920s and 30s including an American chained square vanity case with enamel medallion in centre and a selection of pendant compacts and accessories for necklaces and chatelaines, EPNS compact in the shape of a mirror 1920s with suspension loop; miniature EPNS mirror (oval) with suspension loop; sterling silver locket compact on silver chain; base metal locket compact; solid silver lipstick case with suspension loop and a black plastic compact, set with rhinestones to be worn as brooch or on chatelaine.

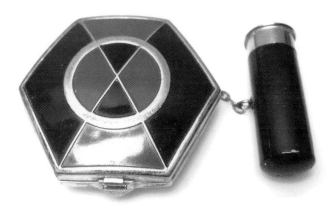

1920s Tango compact, chrome with red and black enamel. *Grays Antiques.*

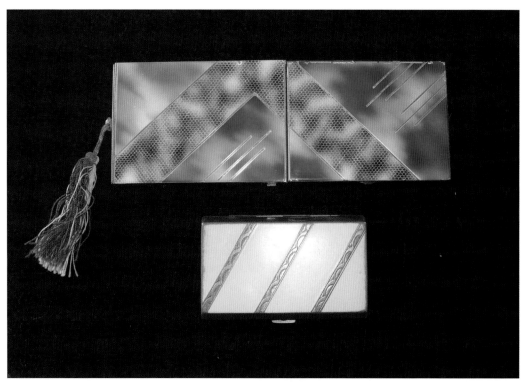

Blue and silver art deco vanity case with compartments for powder, cigarettes and a pull-out lipstick; White and gold art deco vanity case with powder, rouge, lip paste, two eye shadows, mascara and cosmetic pencil.

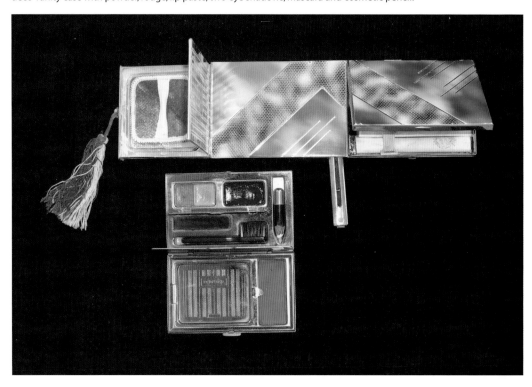

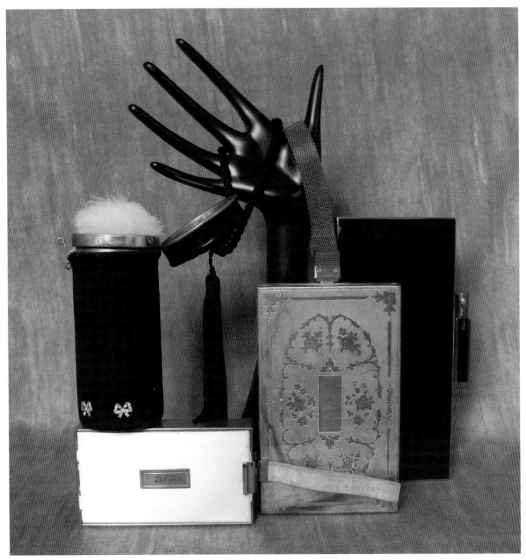

Collection of 1930s carryalls and handbag compacts (left to right) suede-covered tubular vanity case, with powder compact top, silk handle and tassle, made in France; Parklane double sided vanity case, monogrammed DB with metal wrist strap, made in England; large brass minaudiere, made in the USA; black enamel "Beauty-Full" minaudiere, with lipstick catch, made in France.

Compacts were made from every conceivable material, from silver to plastic. In August 1923, Albert Shipton of Birmingham patented a method for decorating painted glass with butterfly wings, which was used to produce jewellery and compacts. The process was costly and labour intensive, and for the cheaper end of the market Gwenda (trade-name of the Birmingham firm Hussey-Dawson) imitated the iridescence of South American butterflies with shiny foil – typical subjects including little Dutch girls, Eighteenth Century-style courting couples, and the crinoline lady, a favourite 1930s image, particularly on dressing table items. Birmingham was the main centre of compact production in the UK and home to the Stratton company, who by the 1930s were making half the compacts used in Britain.

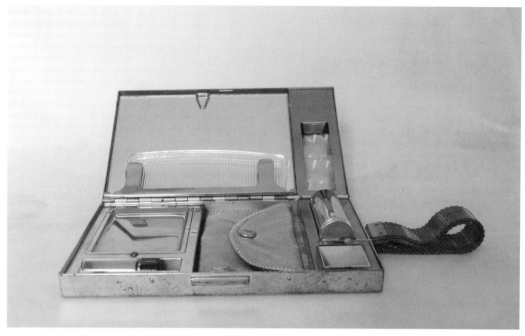

American minaudiere open, showing that some compacts offered more versatility than just powdering the face.

As demand for cosmetics grew, compacts were produced for every pocket. In thirties America, you could spend $6 dollars on a pretty, chain handled Elgin American base metal vanity case or $20 on a similar model in sterling silver. In Britain a Woolworth's compact cost 6d; a Yardley compact two shillings; whilst for anxious husbands searching for a Christmas gift in 1935, *Vogue* recommended an eighteen carat gold minaudiere from Asprey's of London, prices starting at £68 upwards.

Introduced by Paris jewellers Van Cleef and Arpels in 1930, the minaudiere ('pronounced "meen-ode-yair"', advised English *Vogue* helpfully) was the ultimate luxury evening bag. According to company legend, Alfred Van Cleef came up with the idea when, to his horror, he saw a wealthy American client, Florence Jay Gould, bundling away her compact and cosmetics into a common metal container.

Made from gold or platinum and set with gem stones, the minaudiere was a rigid box beautifully fitted with compartments for powder, rouge, lipstick, eye make-up, cigarettes, lighter … everything a femme du monde might need – even noted *Vogue* admiringly 'a little holder for saccharine'. Van Cleef named his new creation after his wife Estelle Arpels, 'qui avait l'habitude de minauder', in other words, who enjoyed making herself charming.

Precious minaudieres were produced by leading jewellers of the day, from Van Cleef and Arpels to Cartier, and more affordable versions of these multi-purpose vanity sets (also known as necessaires and carryalls) became popular across the board. Fitted contents included everything from combs to miniature perfume bottles, and a change purse or coin holder was a useful addition. While men's urinals tended to be free, there was often a charge for visiting women's lavatories. The English phrase 'Spending a penny' derives from the fact that 1d was the standard fee, from the opening of the first public conveniences at the Great Exhibition of 1851, till decimalisation in the 1970s. With the arrival of the powder compact, came another toilet euphemism. Women could now go off 'to powder their noses' and the Ladies became known as the powder room.

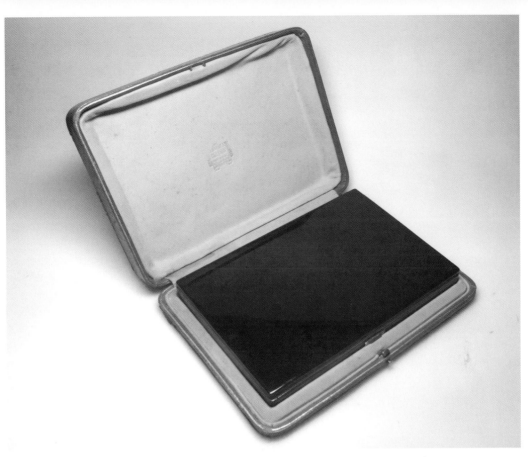

1930s Enamel Minaudiere by Cartier, Paris with gold, diamond and lapis clasp. *Gray's Antiques Market*

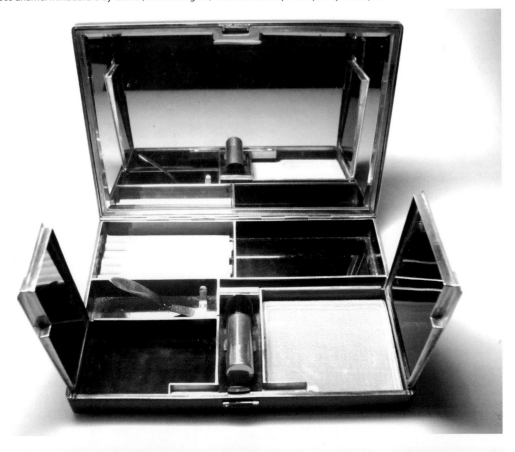

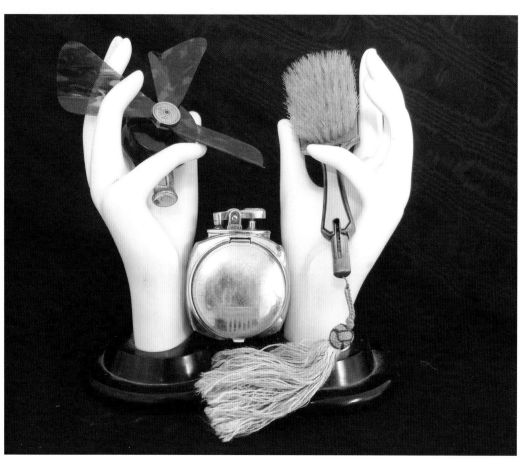

1930s cosmetic novelties: La Brise portable fan with vanity mirror in the back; mauve enamelled hairbrush with pull-out lipstick; Ronson Ladypact combined powder compact and lighter, 1937.

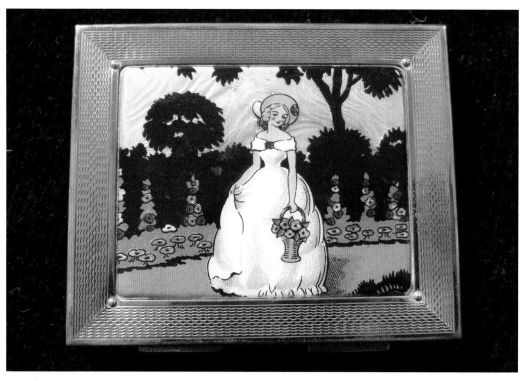

Gwenda compact, 1930s decorated with a foiled picture of a crinoline lady.

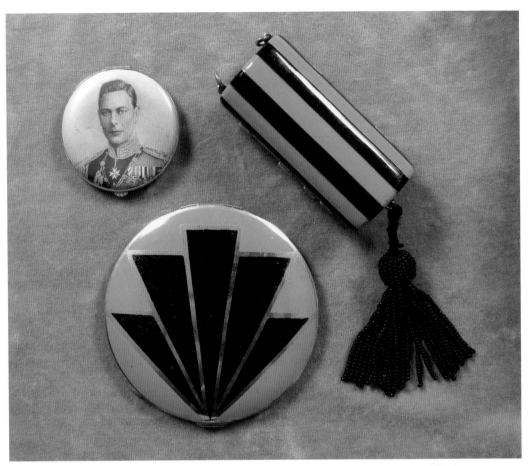

George VI Coronation compact, 1937; Rowenta art deco circular 'flapjack' compact; silver and enamel vanity case with compartments for cosmetics and cigarettes.

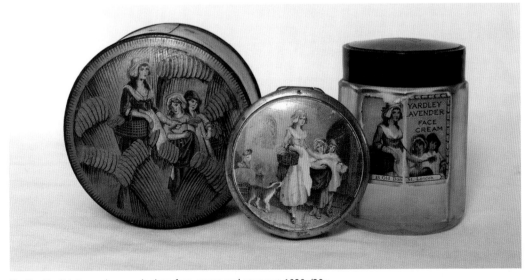

Yardley English Lavender powder box, face cream and compact. 1920s/30s.

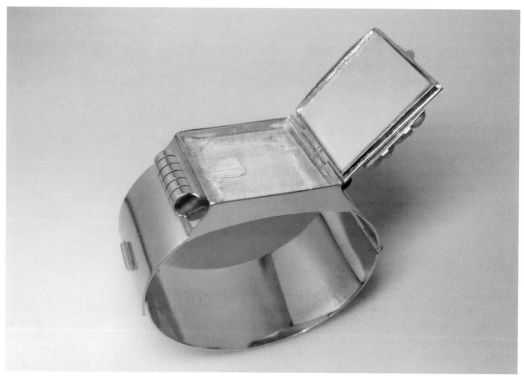

1930s chrome and Bakelite bracelet compact. *Gray's Antiques Market*.

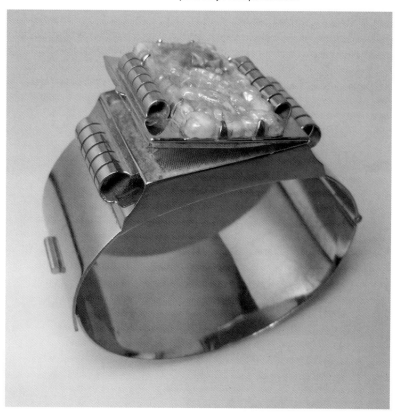

EYE MAKE-UP

"Jeepers Creepers! Where'd ya get those peepers?" asked a famous Johnny Mercer song from the 1930s. The answer was from the wealth of new eye make-up that suddenly appeared on the market. One of the ways eyes appeared that size was thanks to the wealth of make-up and cosmetic aids that were appearing on the market.

The American firm Maybelline pioneered the compact mascara. According to company legend, the product, a mixture of coal dust and Vaseline, was created in 1913 by chemist T.L. Williams for his sister Mabel, whose intended boyfriend had fallen in love with another woman. It worked. Thanks allegedly to her enhanced peepers, Mabel married Chet and in 1915 Williams founded Maybelline, combining his sister's name with Vaseline. Selling initially by mail order, then from 1932 in five and dime stores, priced at an affordable 10c, Maybelline mascara became and remained a brand leader.

Mascara came in cake form with a little brush, the mirrored box providing the one place where it was acceptable (indeed necessary) for a lady to spit. In 1935, English *Vogue* noted the new fashion for liquid mascara – a bottle with a stick applicator – which required a steady hand but was arguably more hygienic.

Germs weren't the only risk when it came to eye make-up. In the 1930s the *Journal of the American Medical Association* reported numerous cases of eye infection, ulceration and worse caused by Lash-Lure, a popular aniline dye for eyebrows and lashes, available in beauty salons across the USA. One woman was permanently blinded when Lash-Lure caused her cornea to fall off, another died from septicemia. Lash-Lure was only one of several damaging products uncovered by the Association during the decade. Anti-Mole, (a remedy containing fifty per cent acid) stripped the skin from the face; a popular freckle ointment caused mercury poisoning; Kromelu depilatory cream was found to be composed largely of rat poison; while those unfortunate enough to dye their hair with Inecto Rapid Notox ended up in hospital with blistered skulls, inflamed faces and a body swollen with pustules. Thanks to Lash-Lure and these other poisonous products, 1938 saw the introduction of the Federal Food, Drug, and Cosmetic Act, which for the first time gave US government the power to regulate cosmetics.

But there were plenty of new make-up accessories to play with which, whilst they might have been a bit tricky to use, at least were unlikely to blind you. In 1916, film director D.W. Griffith is said to have commissioned the first false eyelashes, which were made from human hair woven through gauze for Seena Owen, star of his epic *Intolerance*. Max Factor was one of the pioneering manufacturers and in 1923 Charles (Karl) Nessler (of permanent waving fame) patented a new machine for making false eyelashes, which were supplied by the Nestle company both for theatrical use and everyday wear. Kurlash, the first eyelash curling tongs, were introduced that same year. In the 1930s, *Vogue* advertised eyelash grafting and recommended the new coloured mascaras (blue, green) to set off the latest iridescent eye shadows.

Inspired by stars such as Marlene Dietrich eyebrows were enthusiastically plucked or even shaved off altogether with the new lady razors. They were then drawn in again with an eye pencil (favourite accessory of the period), the arc-shaped lines giving women an air of wide-eyed surprise, that could prove lasting if the hair failed to grow back. Careful grooming was recommended. When Cecil Beaton interviewed Wallis Simpson in 1937, he noted her immaculate appearance, 'she reminds me of the newest, neatest luggage and is as compact as a Louis Vuitton traveling case' her shiny hair 'brushed so that a fly would slip off it' and her 'carefully shaped eyebrows'; which she tidied up with a special little brush kept in her handbag.

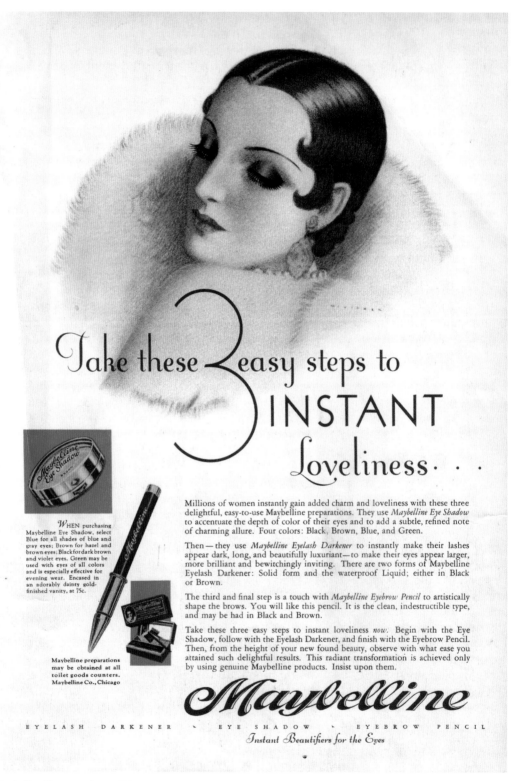

Take these 3 easy steps to

INSTANT

Loveliness · · ·

Millions of women instantly gain added charm and loveliness with these three delightful, easy-to-use Maybelline preparations. They use *Maybelline Eye Shadow* to accentuate the depth of color of their eyes and to add a subtle, refined note of charming allure. Four colors: Black, Brown, Blue, and Green.

Then — they use *Maybelline Eyelash Darkener* to instantly make their lashes appear dark, long, and beautifully luxuriant — to make their eyes appear larger, more brilliant and bewitchingly inviting. There are two forms of Maybelline Eyelash Darkener: Solid form and the waterproof Liquid; either in Black or Brown.

The third and final step is a touch with *Maybelline Eyebrow Pencil* to artistically shape the brows. You will like this pencil. It is the clean, indestructible type, and may be had in Black and Brown.

Take these three easy steps to instant loveliness *now*. Begin with the Eye Shadow, follow with the Eyelash Darkener, and finish with the Eyebrow Pencil. Then, from the height of your new found beauty, observe with what ease you attained such delightful results. This radiant transformation is achieved only by using genuine Maybelline products. Insist upon them.

*W*HEN purchasing Maybelline Eye Shadow, select Blue for all shades of blue and gray eyes; Brown for hazel and brown eyes; Black for dark brown and violet eyes. Green may be used with eyes of all colors and is especially effective for evening wear. Encased in an adorably dainty gold-finished vanity, at 75c.

Maybelline preparations may be obtained at all toilet goods counters. Maybelline Co., Chicago

Maybelline

EYELASH DARKENER · EYE SHADOW · EYEBROW PENCIL
Instant Beautifiers for the Eyes

Maybelline Mascara advert, 1921.

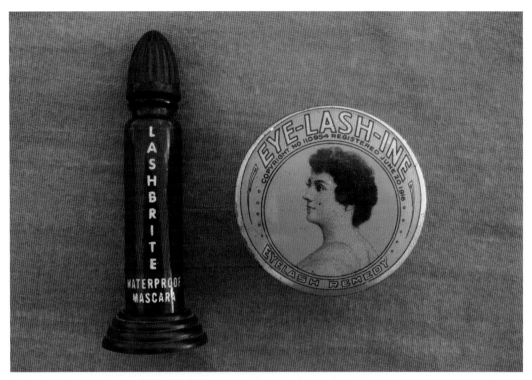

Lashbrite waterproof mascara bottle (1930s); Eye-Lash-Ine eye lash remedy, patented 1916.

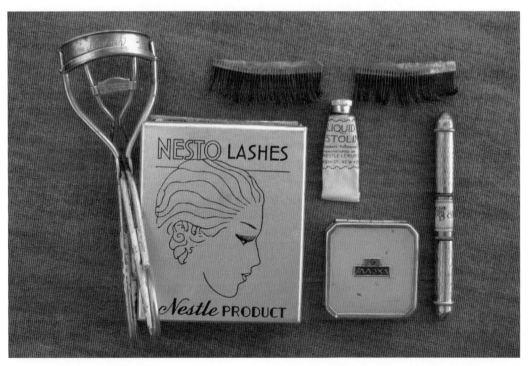

Eye make-up from the 1920s/30s: Nesto false eye lashes; eye pencil by Dorin, Paris; Innoxa eye shadow compact; Kurlash eyelash curler made in the USA.

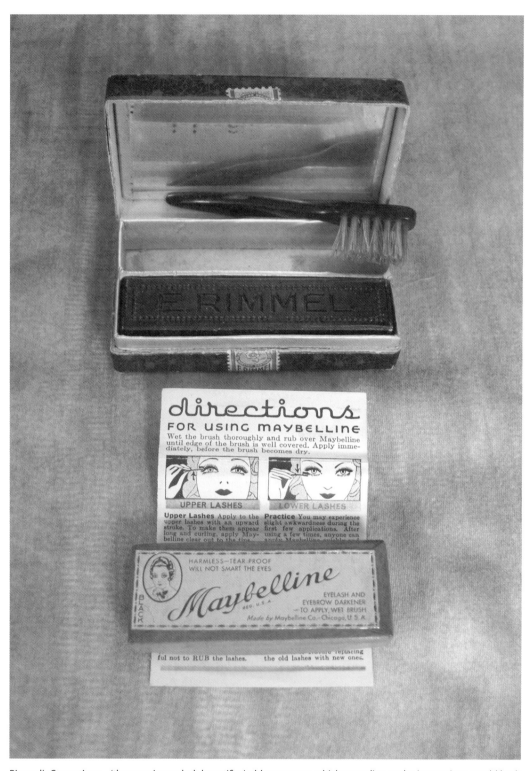

Rimmel's Cosmetique – 'the superior eyelash beautifier' a blue mascara which according to the instructions would both beautify and 'encourage the growth of long languorous lashes'; Maybelline Mascara box, both 1920/30s.

LIPSTICK

In the 1900s, French cosmetic companies such as Bourjois and Guerlain were supplying lip pomade in glass jars and cardboard tubes but it was the Americans who came up with the metal lipstick case that was to become a symbol and favourite handbag accessory of the twenties flapper. In 1915 Maurice Levy designed a simple tube – two inches long with a plain dip-nickel finish and side levers to push up the lipstick – that was produced by the Scovill Manufacturing Company, Connecticut. James Bruce Mason Jr of Nashville, Tennessee patented the now familiar swivel case in 1923 and once lipstick was safely portable and prettily packaged, there was no stopping it.

Tiny lipsticks were made for vanity boxes. Full size enamelled lipsticks were produced in matching sets with powder compacts and cigarette cases. Manufacturers experimented with new opening mechanisms and novelty designs. Engraved silver lipstick cases came with pop-up mirrors; double ended tubes held lipstick at one end and perfume at the other. Fracy 'Allumettes for thy lips' was a little matchbook of disposable lipstick covered sticks, and was supplied in a metal case with mirror. From being something to be used in secret (if at all) the lipstick was now an object to show off in public. In 1934 when Princess Marina married the Duke of Kent wedding gifts included a solid gold lipstick case, set with sapphires and a fold out mirror.

Best-selling brands of the period included Kissproof lipstick and matching rouge ('stays on no matter what one does!' boasted an American advertisement in 1923) and Tangee, made by George W. Luft, New York. Named after tangerine (a classic colour of the tangoing twenties) Tangee natural appeared orange in the tube, went on clear and then promised to blend with your natural colouring. In 1927 French chemist Paul Baudecroux launched 'Rouge Baiser', claiming to be the world's first indelible lipstick and which went on to become a favourite of Audrey Hepburn in the 1950s and a symbol of Parisian sophistication. Louis Philippe (a French émigré who founded his New York cosmetics company in 1911) also offered a bit of continental glamour with his popular Angelus Rouge Incarnat lipstick 'In its allure it is typically, wickedly of Paris. In its virginal modesty, as natural as a jeune fille – ravishing without revealing'.

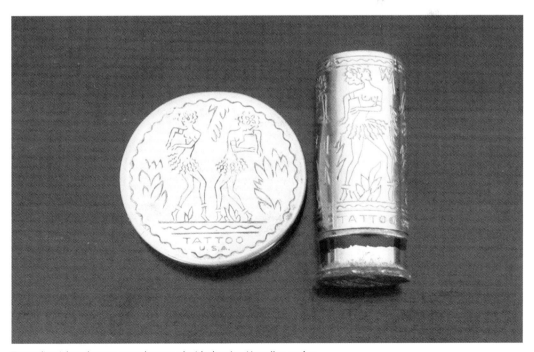

Tattoo lipstick and rouge case decorated with dancing Hawaiian nudes.

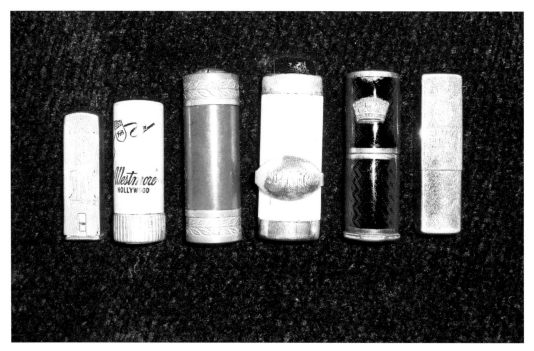

From Left to Right: Art deco lipsticks: silver metal Cutex lipstick; pale green Westmore of Hollywood lipstick; dark green Bakelite and engraved metal lipstick – for Le Rouge Baiser (Paris, France); ridged cream bakelite lipstick with sliding chrome opener, marked Sofistik; blue enamel and silver lipstick with crown crest Elizabeth Arden made by Gieves of London; silver metal rectangular lipstick – Coty Gitane.

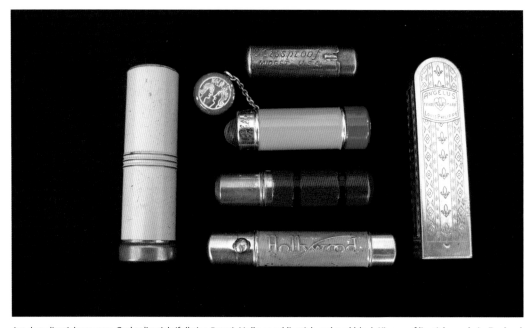

Art deco lipsticks: mauve Cyclax lipstick (full-size 5cms); Hollywood lipstick; red and black Kissproof lipstick, made in England; Helena Rubinstein green Valaze Geranium lipstick with chained and decorated top; engraved brass Kissproof Midget lipstick (3cms) made in the USA; engraved goldtone Louis Philippe Angelus Rouge Incarnat lipstick.

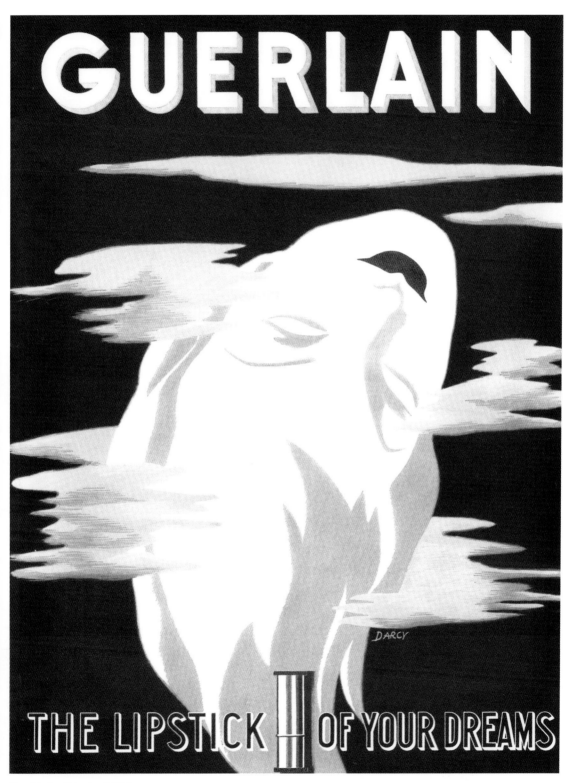

Guerlain lipstick advert, 1930s.

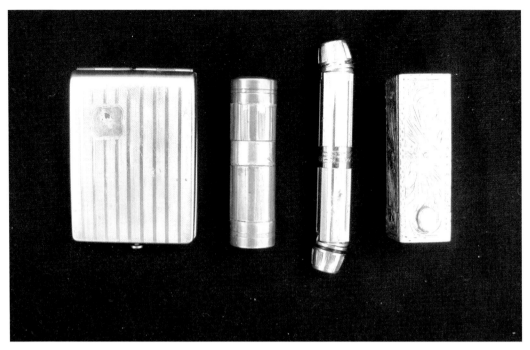

Lipstick novelties closed and open: Fracy lipstick matchbook 'Allumettes for thy lips'; Coty brass lighter in the form of a lipstick tube; Coty double-ended lipstick and perfume atomizer; engraved silver lip-view with pop-up mirror made in Italy.

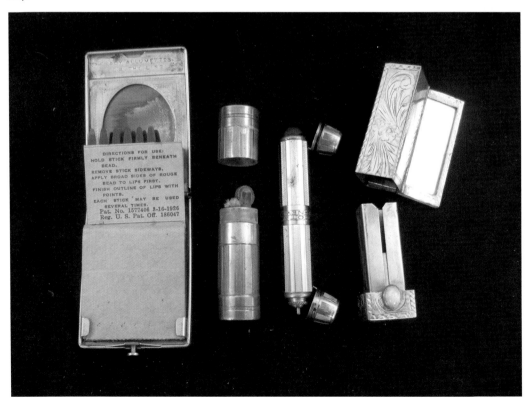

In a world where lipstick was still a comparatively new phenomenon, manufacturers constantly reassured women that lipstick would make them sexy without looking cheap. 'Painted lips are Glaring Lips, Tangee lips are Glowing Lips,' insisted a 1930s advertisement. Some however were less coy. Tussy lipstick by Lesquendieu promised to make you 'Provocative, luscious and gorgeous', while Tattoo lipsticks and compacts were decorated with exotic Hawaian nudes. In 1938 Volupté launched two lipsticks; 'Lady', a light pink shade and the deep red 'Hussy' 'for the girl who "likes to be just a leetle bit shocking"'. Hussy outsold Lady by five to one.

Lipsticks came in an ever-widening range of colours. Schiaparelli created Shocking Pink and Purple Frolic; in English *Vogue* in 1934 society hairdresser Monsieur Antoine (recently arrived from Paris) recommended 'off-black lipstick to be worn by those with the darkest red nails'. Flavoured lipsticks were introduced in the 1920s (cherry was a favourite) and by the 1930s Priscilla Parker was even offering a deodorising lipstick: 'Can you think of a more graceful way to keep your mouth constantly sweet? Kills liquor and cigarette odours.'

HAND CARE
'When we play Bridge (and who doesn't nowadays?) nothing undermines our confidence more than hands which would look better under the table than on it,' claimed *Vogue* in 1934. Whether fanning out cards, opening a compact or cigarette case (period advertisements for nail varnish often illustrated women smoking), a lady's nails were on display and the interwar years saw a remarkable increase in hand care.

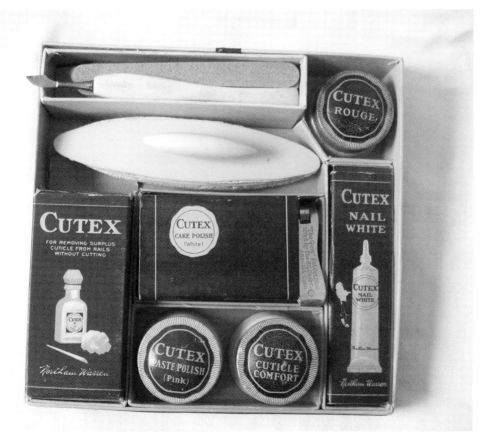

1920s Cutex manicure kit.

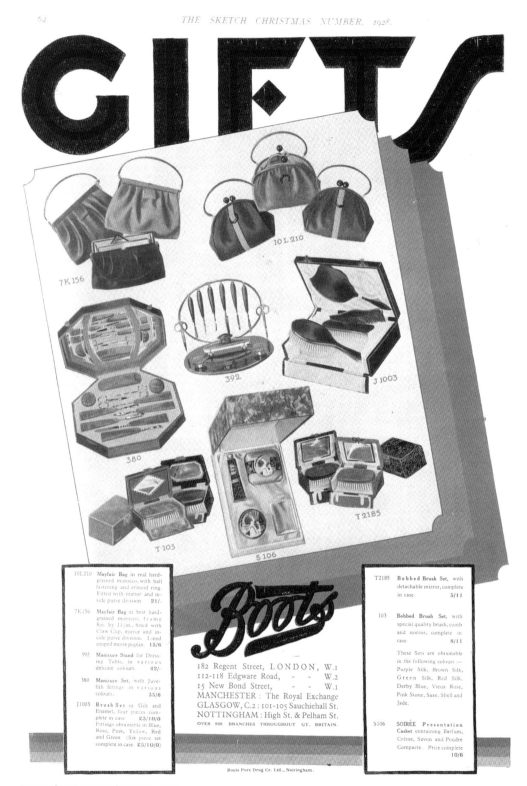

Boots advertisement Christmas, 1928.

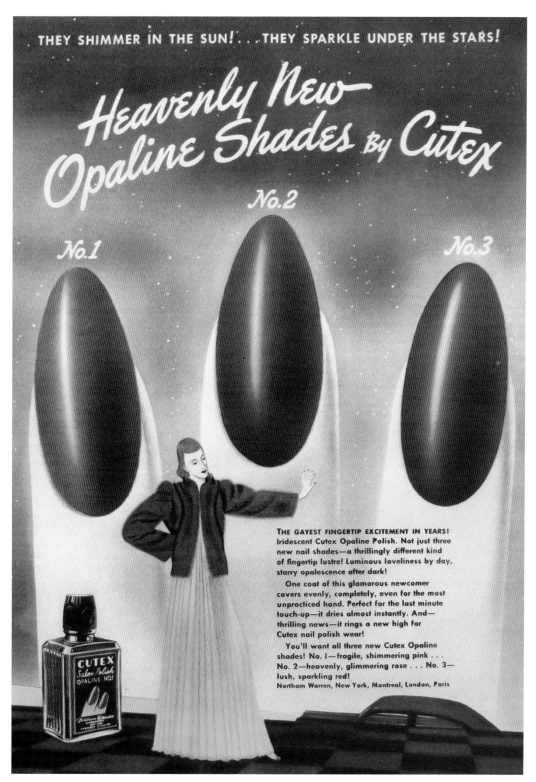

Cutex advertisement, 1940.

In the early twenties only twenty-five per cent of American women manicured their nails, by the 1930s this number had risen to seventy-five per cent. Cutex lured new customers with cheap sample manicure sets advertised in women's magazines. In 1922 a trial box containing 'Cutex cuticle remover, powder polish, cuticle comfort, emery board, orange stick and a little bottle of that marvellous liquid polish that had just been invented' cost only 15c. Having tried it once, women came back for bigger, more expensive kits and according to a Cutex advertisement in December 1937 '8 out of 10 women said we want manicure sets for Christmas'.

The 1920s fashion was for painting the middle of the nail only, leaving the tip and half moon white. Clear nail polishes came in cake and powder form. Paste and liquid varnish provided gentle transparent tints. Nitrocellulose paint however, developed for the burgeoning automobile industry in the early 1920s, created new possibilities. Brothers Charles and Joseph Revson together with Charles Lachman developed an opaque 'cream enamel' that came in a rainbow of vibrant colours. Revlon (the l was for Lachman) was founded in 1932 with only $300 and Charles Revson demonstrated his varnish range to beauty salons by painting each of his own nails in a different shade because it was cheaper than printing a colour chart. A marketing genius, Revson helped transform the nail care industry in the 1930s and 40s. Mirroring the fashion business, he introduced new nail colours every season. Clever advertising and seductive names; Fatal Apple 'the most tempting colour since Eve winked at Adam', Fifth Avenue Red, and Paint the Town Pink, emphasised the fact that he wasn't just selling polish, but romance and fun.

The 1930s saw the fashion for matching lipstick with nail varnish. 'The red of lovely lips is chic … its replica at your fingertips is chic' enticed a 1930s ad for Peggy Sage make-up. Like lipstick, nail polish came in an ever-expanding palette, with colours including blue, green, platinum and even black which, observed Cecil Beaton mockingly in 1937, made 'fingers look as though they had been caught in door lintels'. Traditional pinks and crimsons however remained the most popular colours and with the outbreak of World War II bright red – confident and patriotic – was a favourite choice.

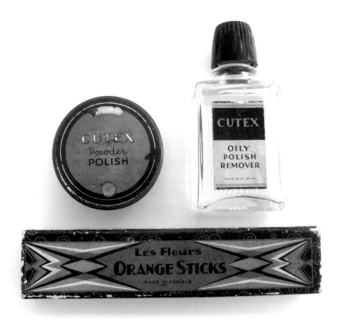

Cutex Powder Polish tin, Cutex Oily Polish Remover bottle, Boots Les Fleurs Orange Sticks, 1920s/30s.

CHAPTER SEVEN

War Paint

Beauty during World War II

'TODAY YOU WANT to look as if you thought less about your face than what you have to face,' announced *Vogue* in 1942 and, for women facing the deprivations of wartime Britain, there was very little choice.

Food rationing began in January 1940, clothing coupons were introduced in June 1941, soap rationing followed eight months later. 'Come in and have a bath rather than a drink, is the new social gesture,' observed *Vogue* at the height of the Blitz, when as people were bombed out of their homes soap, hot water and a bath to enjoy them in became precious commodities. Hair washing was a luxury. *Vogue* recommended once 'every ten days for greasy heads, every three weeks for dry ones,' and when Marlene Dietrich visited Europe to entertain the US troops she took with her three months' supply of dry shampoo.

Cosmetics weren't 'on the ration' but they might just as well have been. In 1940 the Limitation of Supplies Order cut cosmetic production in Britain to just twenty-five per cent of pre-war output. Metal casings were needed for armaments; petroleum, alcohol and other essential beauty ingredients were commandeered for the war effort. Coty manufactured army foot powder and anti-gas ointment alongside make-up. Stratton (who lost four out of their five Birmingham factories to Luftwaffe bombs) converted their lipstick machines to produce shell cases. Gala offered lipstick refills. 'Rescue those old lipstick cases,' encouraged a 1940s ad. 'Saves money, saves metal, helps to win the war and helps you to look beautiful'.

Paper and cardboard were in short supply and make-up (if you were lucky enough to find any) came in utility packaging. Bourjois' Evening in Paris rouge opened up to reveal an emergency note: 'We regret that owing to wartime restrictions PUFFs are unobtainable'. Coty's Air Spun powder was sold in a simple buff coloured container inscribed 'Special War Pack ... identical quality and quantity as the original box'. It might not have looked very pretty, but at least the contents were genuine. Women who turned to the black market ran the risk of returning home with nothing more than a box of powdered chalk.

Paper rationing also caused magazines to reduce in size. Advertising space was severely limited and priority was given to ministry propaganda reminding readers to Dig for Victory, to avoid the Squander Bug, and to invest in war bonds to save the nation: 'Buy nothing for your personal pleasure or comfort ... It is contemptible. To watch every penny shows your will to win' instructed the National Savings Committee in 1940.

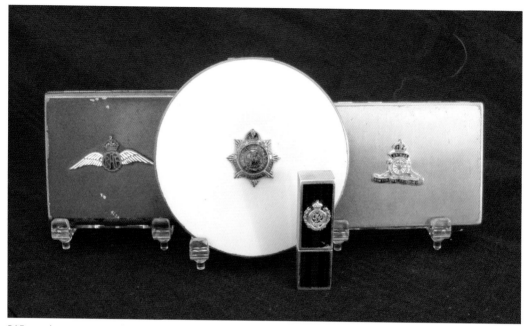

RAF powder compact, made in England; Royal Army Service Corps circular compact, made by Stratton; Royal Engineers silver metal and enamel lipstick; Royal Artillery goldtone compact by Vogue Vanities.

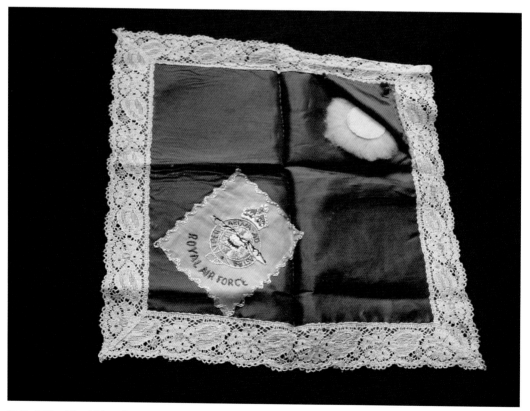

1940s RAF red lipstick handkerchief with an integral powder puff.

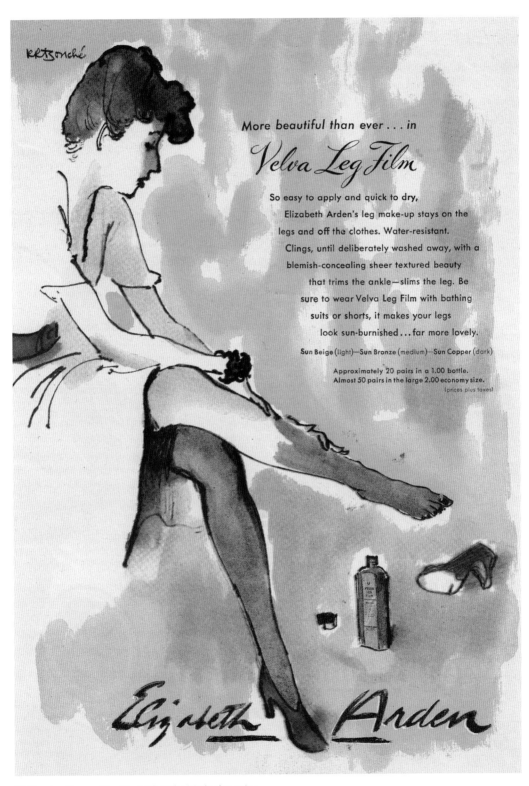

1940s advertisement for Elizabeth Arden's Velva leg paint.

Cosmetic ads, when they did appear, were often apologetic – 'Peggy Sage hopes that her nail polishes will become available in the not too distant future'; 'Elizabeth Arden is anxious as always to help the women of today with their wartime problems, but her salon is strictly rationed'. Manufacturers advised women to use any pre-war cosmetics they had left as sparingly as possible, and offered alternative product-free treatments: 'Hormone Massage … It's the answer to cosmetic shortage,' claimed Helena Rubinstein in 1942, never one to miss a new marketing opportunity even in extremis.

On the one hand simplicity, practicality and rigid economy were the order of the day. 'Il faut skimp pour etre chic,' claimed *Vogue*, 'Dressiness is Démodé'. As women donned uniforms, boiler suits (called siren suits because they could be pulled on as soon as the siren sounded) and utility clothing; so hair and make-up were required to be equally utilitarian. 'Why does that shoulder-mane seem out of date? Because it would look messy hanging on a uniform collar. What's wrong with those exquisite tapered nails? They couldn't do a hand's turn without breaking. Why does that heavy eye make-up seem overdone? Because it would racket with the simplicity of service clothes.' Yet added *Vogue*, 'Nail varnish, like lipstick still looks bravely,' and as women adopted masculine clothes to do men's jobs, how they expressed their femininity became even more important.

Put Your best Face Forward

If you were working in a munitions factory, hair had to be hidden away under hats and headscarves but long Veronica Lake-style tresses could be wound round an old stocking into a victory roll, and even the shorter styles could be home permed into elaborate curls or perhaps dyed peroxide blond, like Jean Harlow.

Hair and make-up were regarded as critical to morale. 'A woman needs cosmetics to look her best, and only when she looks her best can she feel and do her best,' insisted *Vogue* in 1942. 'Cosmetics are as essential to a woman as a reasonable supply of tobacco is to a man,' agreed Mr Henderson from the Ministry of Supply, and according to a munitions factory welfare officer '£1000 worth of cosmetics, distributed among my girls, would please them more than cash'.

In Royal Ordnance factories girls were supplied with foundation and tinted powder to protect them from dermatitis and special cosmetic quotas (particularly lipstick) were set aside for distribution to war workers, although there were never enough to satisfy demand. Women met the shortfall by embracing the same make do and mend attitude that they applied to their clothes. Beetroot juice served for lipstick and boot polish for mascara. *Good Housekeeping* magazine suggested rubbing the face with cucumber or a piece of apple as a DIY astringent and using a flour and water paste to discipline unruly eyebrows. Margarine and milk powder boiled in water made an austerity face cream.

The other option was buying either under the counter or on the black market, where women looked not just for make-up but for that other most wanted wartime fashion commodity – a pair of silk or even nylon stockings. With the declaration of war, it was impossible to import silk from major producers Japan, Italy and China. The manufacture of silk stockings was banned in Britain in 1941 and in the US the government commandeered the national supply of silk to be transformed into cartridge bags. Nylons had only just emerged before the war and in 1942 American women were asked not only to hand in their silk stockings for recycling but also their nylons, which were melted down and remade into parachutes. The stocking alternatives were wool, rayon or one of the few new cosmetic inventions to emerge during the war, leg paint.

For those lucky enough to get hold of it 'liquid stocking' was produced by firms including Elizabeth Arden, Max Factor and Cyclax. For the majority of British girls who couldn't, one option was painting the legs with tea or gravy browning, and getting a friend with an eye pencil and a very steady hand to draw a seam down the back.

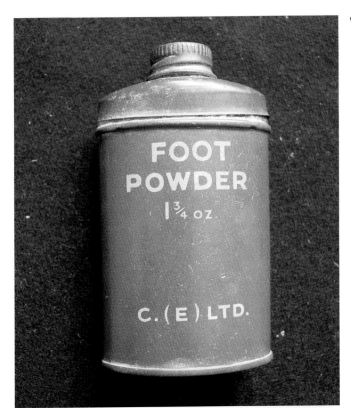

World War Two tin of Army Foot Powder.

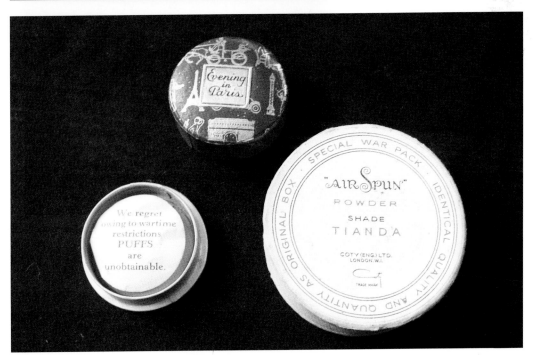

World War Two Utility Packaging – Bourjois Evening in Paris rouge and Coty Air Spun powder inscribed 'Special War Pack'.

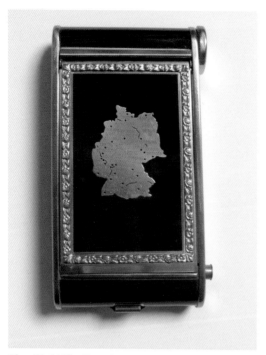

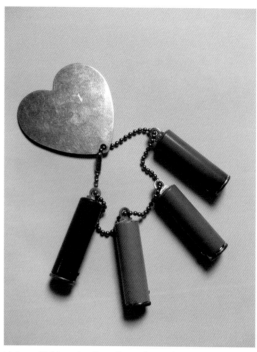

After World War Two, Germany was divided into zones occupied by the Allies. This compact is decorated with a map showing the US zone. Goldtone and tortoiseshell enamel, made in Germany.

Helena Rubinstein Four-Cast charm bracelet with four different coloured lipsticks and heart shaped metal mirror, 1940s.

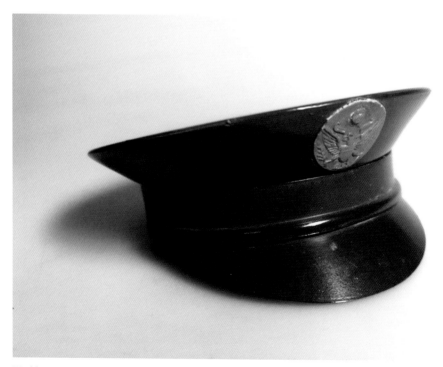

World War Two plastic compact in the shape of US army officer's cap, early 1940s.

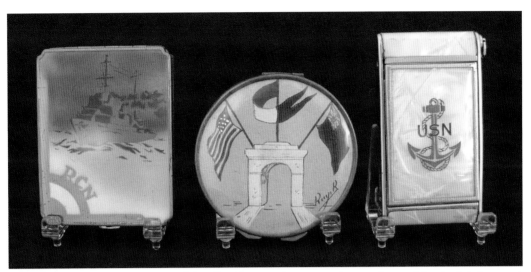

World War Two powder compacts: Royal Canadian Navy powder compact brass and enamel; hand painted compact celebrating the liberation of France and showing American, French and Canadian flags; US Navy chrome and plastic mother of pearl vanity case made by Zell.

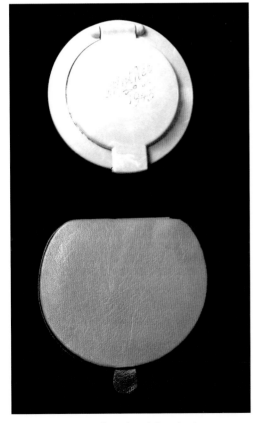

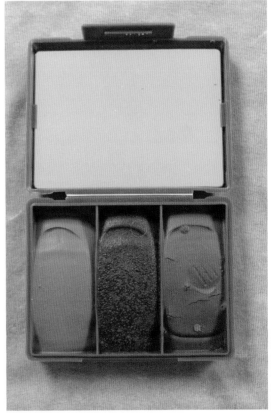

World War Two cardboard and faux leather compact using no metal parts; all-plastic compact, hand engraved Mother 1945 and containing a Pond's Angel Face powder puff.

Contemporary Camouflage face paint compact, similar to those produced for the armed forces during World War Two.

American servicemen – famously overpaid, over-sexed and over here – provided a welcome supply of rationed goods and a powder compact designed for one of the US or Canadian Armed forces was a coveted status symbol. Around 1.5 million American GIs (so called because their equipment was labelled government issue) passed through Britain during the war years, bringing with them their slang, their jitterbugging, and their consumer luxuries: gum, real coffee, tinned peaches, scented soap, and a bit of much needed glamour. For British women they were not just a potential source of cosmetics and stockings, but a reason to wear them. 'So many nice lads – Norwegian, Polish, Canadian and of course the GIs. We all made dates that we could never possibly keep and had the time of our lives, never expecting the war could be such fun,' remembered one London girl. 'There was no question of settling down with anyone, just the sheer enjoyment of dancing with soldiers of different nationalities in different styles. We re-cut our mothers' dance dresses, wore as much make-up as we could, and loved every minute.'

Over 80,000 British girls did in fact 'settle down' and ended up as GI Brides but it wasn't just single girls on the pull who piled on the slap. 'How do you look when he comes home?' demanded a 1942 article in *Good Housekeeping*. Not 'letting yourself go – taking time to powder your nose and redden your lips,' was seen as important to a husband's morale when he was involved in war work and was portrayed part as of a English woman's patriotic duty.

Arian Purity

In Germany, it was different. When the fascist division of the Mitford sisters (Diana and Unity) visited the Fuhrer in the thirties, his aids referred to them as painted hussies –

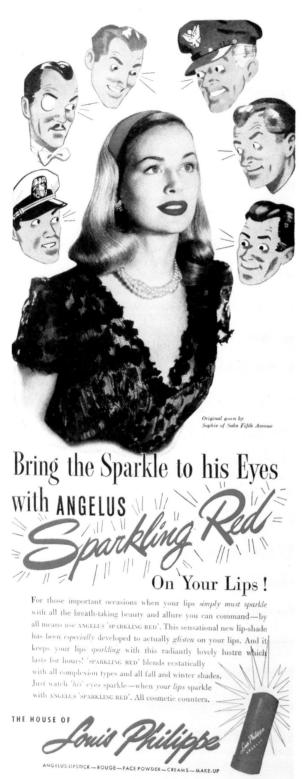

Bring the Sparkle to his Eyes with ANGELUS *Sparkling Red* On Your Lips !

For those important occasions when your lips *simply must sparkle* with all the breath-taking beauty and allure you can command—by all means use ANGELUS 'SPARKLING RED'. This sensational new lip-shade has been *especially* developed to actually *glisten* on your lips. And it keeps your lips *sparkling* with this radiantly lovely lustre which lasts for hours! 'SPARKLING RED' blends ecstatically with all complexion types and all fall and winter shades. Just watch '*his*' eyes sparkle—when *your* lips sparkle with ANGELUS 'SPARKLING RED'. All cosmetic counters.

THE HOUSE OF *Louis Philippe*

ANGELUS LIPSTICK—ROUGE—FACE POWDER—CREAMS—MAKE-UP

1945 advertisement for Louis Philippe Angelus Sparkling Red lipstick, showing a girl attracting the attention of service men.

because of their lipstick and eye make-up – and they were booed in the street. Hitler disliked lipstick, claiming it was made of animal fats extracted from sewage. The precise list of instructions issued to visitors at Berchtesgaden (his mountain retreat) restricted both smoking and make-up: 'Women guests are forbidden to use excessive cosmetics and must on no account use colouring material on their fingernails.' The Arian ideal was a clean scrubbed face and, with the notable exception of Eva Braun whose personal effects included silver monogrammed compacts, cigarette cases and lip views, women of the Third Reich were expected to eschew drinking, smoking, and cosmetics.

Lipstick – The Red Badge of Courage

In Britain make-up might have been hard to find but it was worn with pride and became a symbol of the will to win. 'Put your best face forward,' encouraged a 1942 Yardley advertisement in Churchillian tones, 'We have to remember that to yield to carelessness is to lower our standard to the enemy. There must be no surrender to circumstances, no giving ground to careless grooming … Never should we forget that good looks and good morale go hand in hand.'

'England expects these days that every woman shall be a beauty,' agreed a 1940s ad for Tattoo lipstick. 'War, Woman and lipstick,' ran a celebrated Tangee campaign. Bright red was the favourite wartime colour for lips and nails and lipstick names were often patriotic: Louis Philippe's 'Patriot Red', 'Fighting Red' by Tussy and 'Grenadier … The new Military red created by Tattoo – effective with navy or air force blue, and khaki.'

British and American cosmetic advertise-ments featured girls in uniform and factory overalls, boldly sporting bright lipstick ('Will help you to be attractive as well as efficient,' promised Tangee) or dressed in their best civvies and beautifully made up to greet their returning servicemen sweethearts. A typical 1944 ad for Tussy skin creams showed a kissing couple under the banner headline 'The Girl Who Landed a Pilot'.

During wartime a subtle change had taken place in the marketing and the perception of make-up. It was no longer about making a woman seem 'dainty' but making her look and feel strong.

Rosie the Riveter became a wartime icon in the USA, representing the six million women working in factories for the war effort. The fictional folk heroine appeared in songs, films and posters and was famously painted by Norman Rockwell for the May 1943 edition of the *Saturday Evening Post*. Rockwell portrayed Rosie as a vast figure in work dungarees, her short sleeves revealing arms the size of prize-winning hams as she eats a sandwich. Behind her hangs the Stars and Stripes, squashed carelessly under her feet is copy of Adolf Hitler's *Mein Kampf*, and on her mighty lap rests a tin lunch box and a huge phallic riveting machine like an enormous gun. On the one hand Rosie is the epitome of butch, but her henna red curls, lipsticked mouth and painted finger nails stress her femininity, emphasising the fact that make-up too was a weapon of war.

Gunpowder and Camouflage make-up

Cosmetics manufacturers also played a more explicit part in the war effort. Charles Revson received an Army and Navy award for manufacturing munitions; a contract which according to his biographer Andrew Tobias he allegedly won by mistake. When a government official asked him if he knew anything about powder (meaning gunpowder) Revson (thinking face powder) replied simply, 'Everything,' and found himself producing hand grenades.

Elizabeth Arden, Helena Rubinstein and Max Factor developed cosmetics for the armed forces. Max Factor created coloured camouflage make-up for the US Marines including jungle green, sand yellow, and night black. For Operation Torch, the British/American invasion of French North Africa that started in November 1942, Helena Rubinstein supplied US troops with customised make-up boxes including cleanser, sunburn cream and camouflage cosmetics for desert conditions. In America, Elizabeth Arden was commissioned to boost the morale of the American Marine Corps

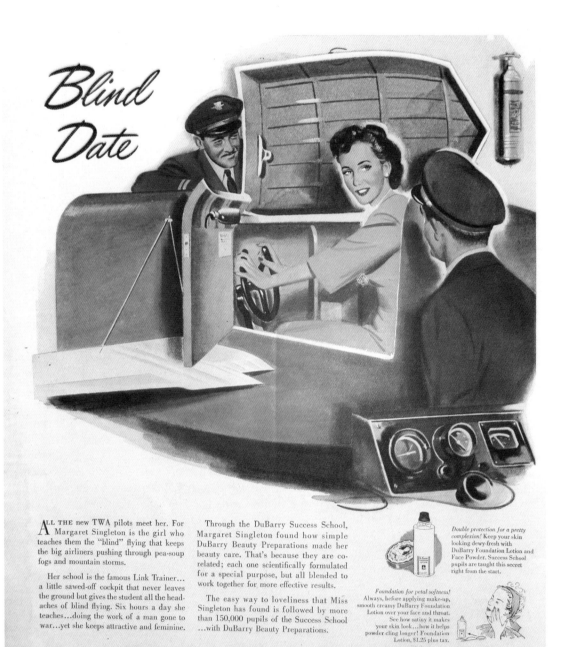

Blind Date

ALL THE new TWA pilots meet her. For Margaret Singleton is the girl who teaches them the "blind" flying that keeps the big airliners pushing through pea-soup fogs and mountain storms.

Her school is the famous Link Trainer... a little sawed-off cockpit that never leaves the ground but gives the student all the headaches of blind flying. Six hours a day she teaches...doing the work of a man gone to war...yet she keeps attractive and feminine.

Through the DuBarry Success School, Margaret Singleton found how simple DuBarry Beauty Preparations made her beauty care. That's because they are co-related; each one scientifically formulated for a special purpose, but all blended to work together for more effective results.

The easy way to loveliness that Miss Singleton has found is followed by more than 150,000 pupils of the Success School ...with DuBarry Beauty Preparations.

Double protection for a pretty complexion! Keep your skin looking dewy-fresh with DuBarry Foundation Lotion and Face Powder. Success School pupils are taught this secret right from the start.

Foundation for petal softness! Always, before applying make-up, smooth creamy DuBarry Foundation Lotion over your face and throat. See how satiny it makes your skin look...how it helps powder cling longer! Foundation Lotion, $1.25 plus tax.

Finishing touch for flattery. DuBarry Face Powder lights up natural skin tones, gives such a wonderful, smooth look. Its glamorous protection lasts for hours. Face Powder, $1.00 and $2.00, plus tax.

Du BARRY
BEAUTY PREPARATIONS
by RICHARD HUDNUT

*Featured in the Richard Hudnut Salon and DuBarry Success School
693 Fifth Avenue, New York 22, N.Y....and at better cosmetic counters everywhere*

Blind Date – World War Two advertisement for Du Barry Beauty Preparations – featuring pilot instructor Margaret Singleton 'Doing the work of a man gone to war … yet she keeps attractive and feminine,' 1944.

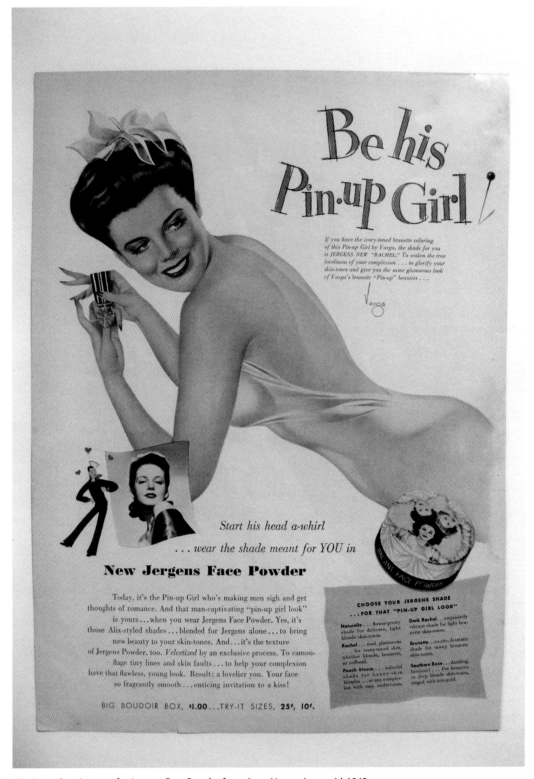

Wartime advertisement for Jergens Face Powder featuring a Varga pin-up girl, 1943.

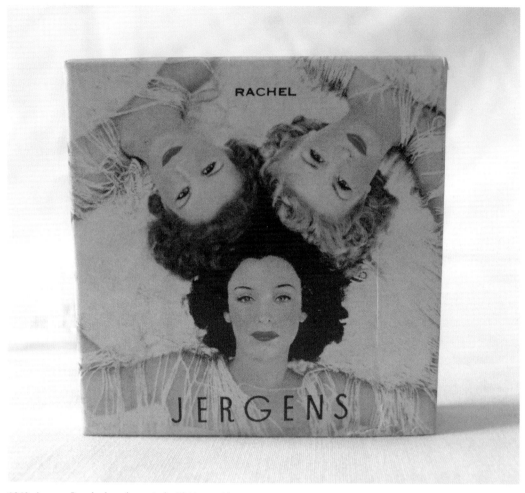

1940s Jergens Powder box decorated with Varga girls.

Women's Reserve, with a make-up kit composed of rouge, lipstick and nail varnish. She matched the colour to the chevrons on their uniform and called it Montezuma red.

In London Miss Arden's British chemists worked with Sir Harold Delf Gillies, the founding father of modern plastic surgery, to create a tinted scar cream to help conceal burns and other wartime injuries.

Providing camouflage on the battlefield, cosmetic surgery in hospital, and general morale boosting on the home front, make-up fulfilled a very serious function during wartime, without ever losing its essential glamour. Rosie the Riveter wasn't the only pin-up of the period. The term 'pin-up' itself emerged in the early forties as servicemen cut out their favourite girly pictures from magazines and pasted or pinned them up in their quarters. Famous pin-ups of the period ranged from Hollywood stars: Betty Grable, with her million dollar legs; Jane Russell with her cantilevered bra (allegedly designed by Howard Hughes); to cartoon cheesecake such as the Petty Girl and the Varga girl, named respectively after George Petty and Alberto Vargas, the illustrators who created them.

Whether real or imaginary what these girls tended to have in common was great legs, magnificent breasts and an encouraging smile. Though their role was often to wear as few

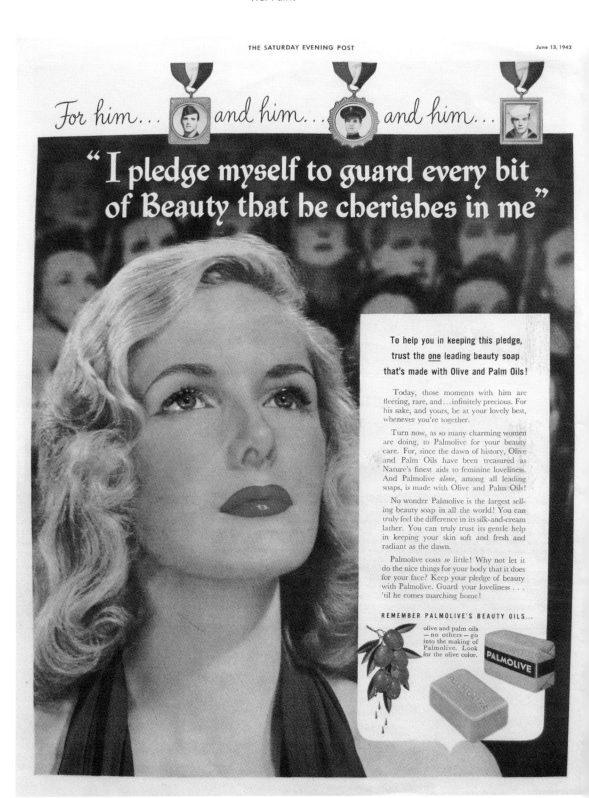

US Palmolive Soap advertisement, 1942.

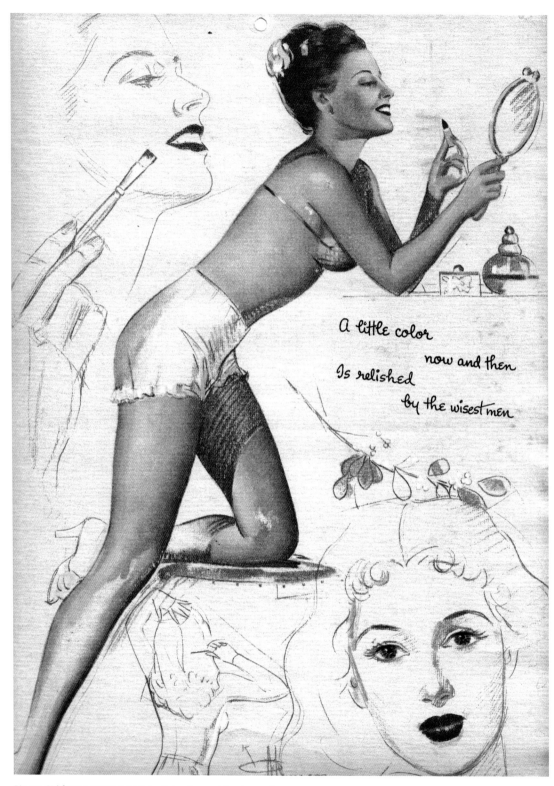

A little color
now and then
Is relished
by the wisest men

Pin-up Girl from a 1940s American Calendar applying her make-up.

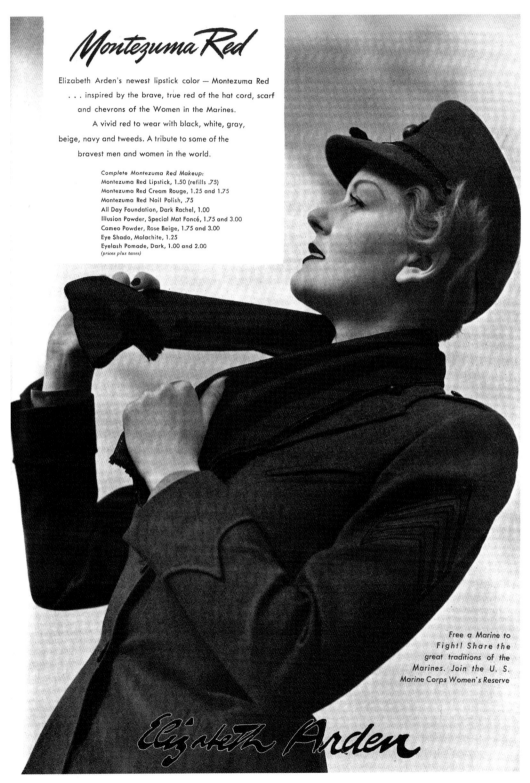

Montezuma Red

Elizabeth Arden's newest lipstick color — Montezuma Red
. . . inspired by the brave, true red of the hat cord, scarf
and chevrons of the Women in the Marines.

A vivid red to wear with black, white, gray,
beige, navy and tweeds. A tribute to some of the
bravest men and women in the world.

Complete Montezuma Red Makeup:
Montezuma Red Lipstick, 1.50 (refills .75)
Montezuma Red Cream Rouge, 1.25 and 1.75
Montezuma Red Nail Polish, .75
All Day Foundation, Dark Rachel, 1.00
Illusion Powder, Special Mat Foncé, 1.75 and 3.00
Cameo Powder, Rose Beige, 1.75 and 3.00
Eye Shado, Malachite, 1.25
Eyelash Pomade, Dark, 1.00 and 2.00
(prices plus taxes)

Free a Marine to
Fight! Share the
great traditions of the
Marines. Join the U. S.
Marine Corps Women's Reserve

Elizabeth Arden

Elizabeth Arden advertisement for Montezuma Red make-up, 1940s.

clothes as printably possible you would never catch them without lipstick and nail varnish. With their generous curves and immaculate hair and make-up the pin-ups of the forties provided an escape from the masculine rigours of war and presaged the return of femininity in the fabulous, frivolous fifties.

The Austerity Dressing Table

At the outbreak of war, powder compacts decorated with British armed forces insignia were produced for service women and men who wanted a gift for the girls back home. Designs were often simple: a plain enamelled compact with a metal badge or regimental transfer applied to the centre. As the conflict continued however metal became increasingly precious. Housewives were encouraged to give 'Saucepans for Spitfires' and donate metal-ware to scrap drives; iron railings disappeared overnight from parks and gardens; and with the enforcement of emergency restrictions, the manufacture of metal compacts ceased in 1942 and wasn't resumed in Britain until after the war.

Replacement compacts were produced in plastic and cardboard, carefully designed to use no metal parts even in the hinges. Make-up came in undecorated emergency packaging and, with supplies being reduced by seventy-five per cent, women had to use their initiative. If you claimed to be an actress, you were entitled to a special allowance of theatrical greasepaint. Buying under the counter was an option and some local chemists produced their own cosmetics disguised as medical products. Women dug out their grandmother's recipes for making DIY soaps and lotions; a favourite Christmas present was a home-made powder puff, sewn from rabbit fur.

Across the Atlantic, US cosmetic firms produced patriotic vanity cases enamelled in red, white and blue and handsome compacts were designed for the US armed forces. As in Europe, the American people were encouraged to save and salvage. A decree, passed in 1942, stipulated that hair cut off in beauty parlours should be collected and recycled into thread for textiles. Cardboard replaced metal lipstick tubes and a popular novelty compact came in the shape of a uniform hat, produced in different colours and with relevant cap badge, for the various US services, and made entirely from plastic.

Shortages might have lead to recycling and reduced packaging, but having tried and failed to limit supplies of beauty products in 1942 the United States War Production Board declared cosmetics to be 'necessary and vital' to the war effort. Dorothy Gray's 'All Clear Red' lipstick was launched that same year.

Government funded research led to new products. A portable insect spray developed for US troops in 1943 to combat malaria-spreading bugs resulted in the creation of the modern aerosol can and the post war hairspray. Emergency restrictions inspired streamlined, economical production methods and improved distribution techniques that, once war was over, would help confirm the United States as the world's leading manufacturer and exporter of beauty products.

CHAPTER EIGHT

Immaculate Grooming

Beauty in the 1940s and 1950s

AFTER THE RIGOURS of war women were desperate for a bit of fun and frivolity, but in Britain they had to wait. The United Kingdom was on the verge of bankruptcy, crippled by wartime debt of $3.5 million to the USA. Abroad the British Empire was being dismantled, at home half a million houses had been destroyed by the Blitz. Millions were living in slums or prefabs, and there was a pressing need for reconstruction and the creation of the welfare state.

With little money to build this brave new world, emergency restrictions remained enforced. Luxury goods were produced for export only. Women who wanted a pair of nylons or some French cosmetics had to resort to the black market. The spiv (suggested origins of his name ranging from VIPs backwards, to spiffy – a Victorian word for smart) became a familiar post-war figure. Presiding over a suitcase full of goodies in his double-breasted camel coat, his padded-shouldered American style suit and kipper dazzle tie, he was certainly one of the few well-dressed figures in austerity Britain.

Shortages were worse than during the war. The allocation of clothing coupons was reduced and for the first time bread was put on the ration. Even the weather contributed to the gloom. Early 1947 saw the severest winter in 300 years and things in Britain were at their very worst when in France a young fashion designer launched his first ever collection.

The New Look
'This Season's sensation is the new house of Christian Dior,' thrilled *Vogue*; 'Paris is more feminine than ever. Paris rounds every line,' enthused *Harper's Bazaar*. To a world starved of ladylike glamour what became known as Dior's New Look was a revelation: beautifully padded jackets that emphasised the bust and flared out over the hips; waist-whittling corsetry and most shocking of all, long, flowing skirts using yards of precious rationed material. 'I designed clothes for flower-like women,' claimed Dior, 'I revived the neglected art of pleasing.' But initially he created a scandal. In Paris a Dior model had a dress ripped from her back, in London politicians campaigned against this outrageous waste of fabric, in America protestors brandished placards saying 'Burn M. Dior'. But women loved this new feminine style, soon everybody was wearing circle skirts supported by layers of frothy nylon petticoats, and Dior's hourglass silhouette became the look of the 1950s.

"Fashion plate"

Cream Wafer Face Make-Up by REVLON

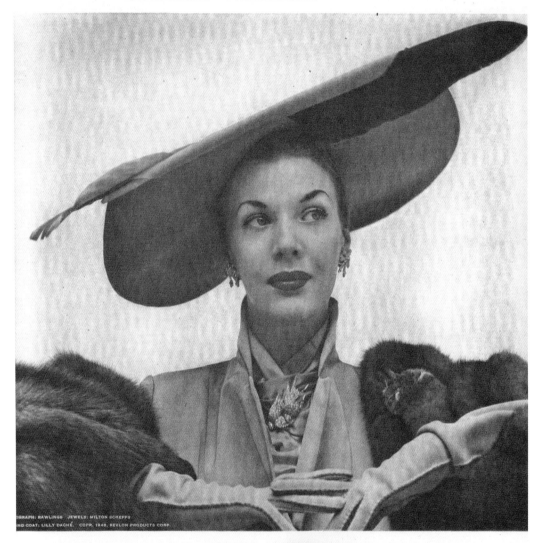

IT'S GOING PLACES . . . in the smartest handbags! It's *designed* to keep the poreless-as-porcelain perfection of the "Fashion Plate" complexion . . . at your fingertips . . . always.

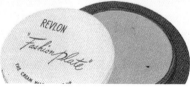

JUST FINGER-STROKE IT ON . Not a cake, "Fashion Plate" needs water or sponge. It *ends* the old-fashioned, dry, mask-y look! Choo from exclusive fashion-genius cold

Revlon Fashion Plate advertisement, 1949.

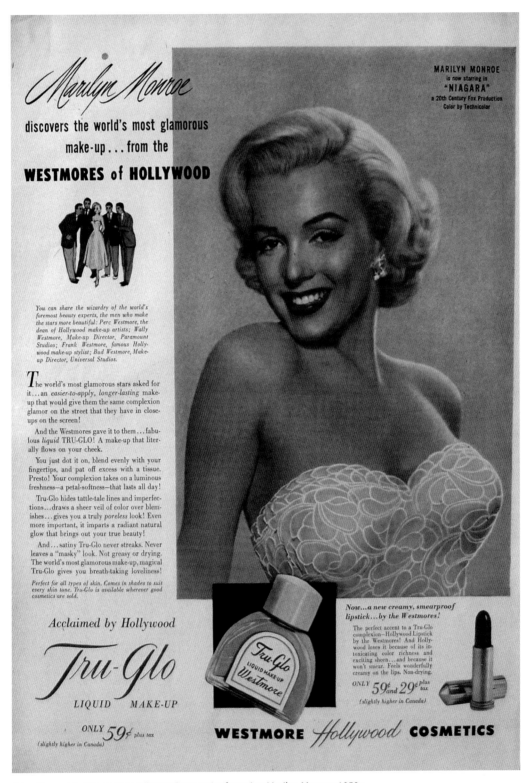

Advertisment for Westmore Hollywood cosmetics featuring Marilyn Monroe, 1950s.

The Curvaceous Fifties

Much as the boyish flat-chested flapper of the twenties replaced the the S-shaped full-breasted Edwardian lady, so the sharp, skimpy silhouette of wartime utility fashion was swept away by the voluptuous curves of fifties style. Marilyn Monroe, Jayne Mansfield, Betty Page, Sophia Loren; fifties stars were notably hour-glass shaped and made the most of their assets. Marilyn's bra size was

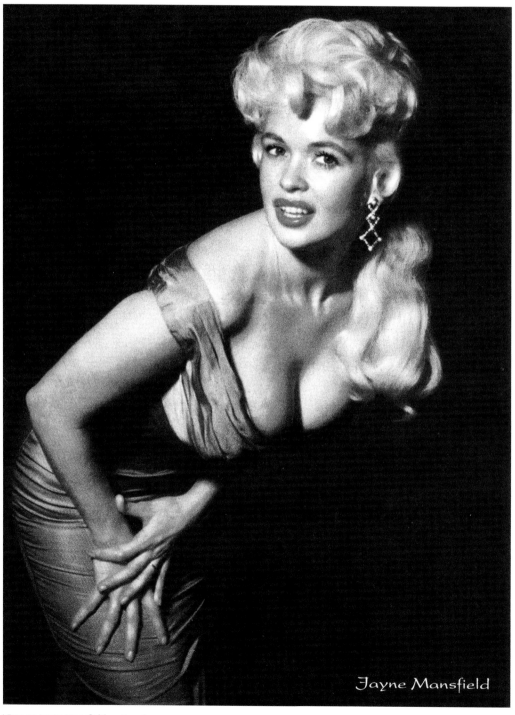

Vintage Jayne Mansfield postcard.

allegedly 36D, Jayne Mansfield described herself as having 36in hips, an 18in waist and a 44D bust. Admittedly very few women could aspire to such magnificent proportions, but what nature couldn't supply new developments in underwear could. Breasts were thrust outwards, with pointing, circle-stitch 'sweater girl' bras; the waist was pulled in with a 'waspie' corset; the stomach flattened and the hips shaped by the latest nylon girdles, supporting the sheerest nylon stockings.

Not since the Edwardian period had women worn such viciously controlling accessories. Ladies tortured their feet with stiletto heels and winkle-picker toes. Evening gowns came with sharply boned bodices designed to maximise feminine curves.

During the war women had done male jobs and worn masculine style uniforms. Once their men were demobbed women were back into the kitchen to await the end of rationing, back into the bedroom to create the baby boom, (much needed to ensure the wealth of the new Elizabethan age) and back into ultra-feminine fashions and make-up.

The Flawless Face

Cosmetics were crucial for obtaining this new ladylike look. The first thing a lady needed was a perfect (or at least perfect-looking) complexion. Cream powder was preferred by many women to loose powder. Max Factor's Pan-Cake – applied with a damp sponge and advertised by all the leading stars of the day – was a best-seller from the 1940s 'gives you a glamorous new complexion … soft, smooth as a pearl and flawless'. In 1948 the company launched Pan-Stik, a cream foundation in stick form, housed in a twist-up, lipstick-style plastic container that could be slipped into a handbag.

This flawless base (which could look very peculiar if you didn't remember to extend it over your décolletage) provided a perfect backdrop for elaborate decoration. In a period that prized the sensual, full-bodied woman, lips were all important. Colours were strong and shiny – fuchsia pink, bright coral, dark red. In 1950 US cosmetic chemist Hazel Bishop (1906-98) launched her famous smear-proof Long-Lasting Lipstick. 'Stays on you … not on him,' boasted the publicity. Within three years her company had captured twenty-five per cent of the American lipstick market with sales of over $10 million.

Whereas lipstick advertisements during the war had stressed courage and resilience, now they sold sex. In his 1949 poster for Rouge Baiser artist René Gruau (1909-2004) wrapped an elegant lady in a blindfold that not only emphasised her scarlet mouth but also carried distinctly erotic overtones. To a public still battling with post-war shortages, this sophisticated, sexy image encapsulated the notion of Parisian chic and helped confirm Rouge Baiser as an iconic French brand.

'Are you made for Fire and Ice?' demanded Revlon in 1952, launching not just a fiery red lipstick and nail polish but another famous cosmetic campaign.

Charles Revson was characteristically forthright about the type of models he wanted for the promotion: 'Park Avenue whores – elegant but with the sexual thing underneath.' The double spread advertisement featured on one page, model Dorian Leigh, in a figure-hugging sliver-sequined evening dress, scarlet-tipped fingers playing over her panting, scarlet-lipped mouth and on the other side, a tick box questionnaire. 'Do you blush when you find yourself flirting? Have you ever wanted to wear an ankle bracelet? Do you close your eyes when you're kissed?' If you answered yes to at least eight of the fifteen questions then, promised the copy, you were ready for 'Fire and Ice'. As Revlon executives explained, the aim of the ads was to show 'There's a little bit of bad in every good woman,' and lipstick would help you unleash it.

Luscious lips were a feature of every icon of the period from Monroe to Mansfield, but this was a controlled, glamorous, sexuality and they had to be perfectly painted. Gala Lip Line (introduced c.1948) was slim as a pencil and recommended for outlining the lips. For the true perfectionist, there was the Hollywood 'Glamour Lips' applicator – a metal contraption in the shape of a Cupid's

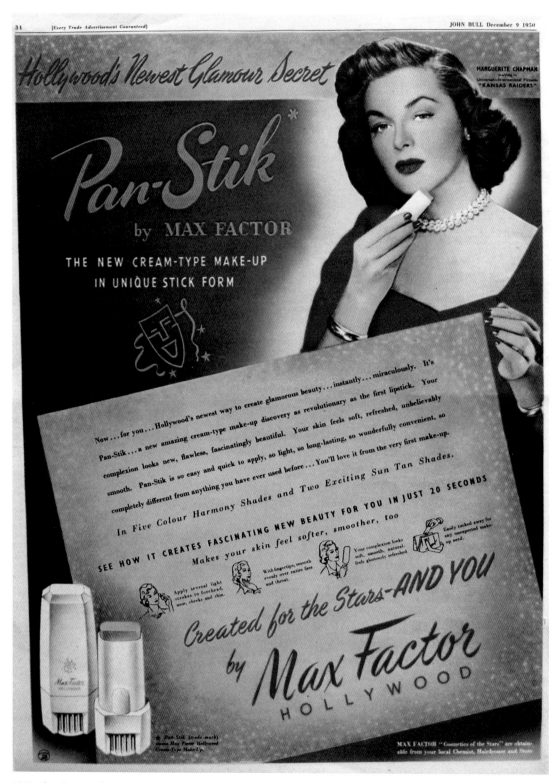

1950 advertisement for Max Factor Pan-Stik.

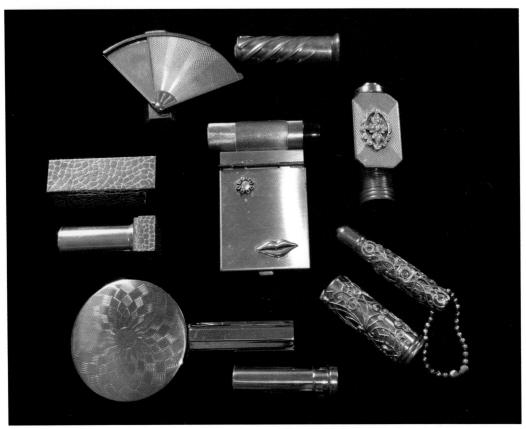

1950s lipstick and lip-views. Clockwise from top: Stratton lip-view with fan-shaped sliding mirror; Yardley lipstick with blue plastic bee set in top; Fortuna pop-up lip-view with marcasite decoration; Rimmel jewelled lipstick with matching miniature pen in jeweled case with chain; Stratton folding lipstick mirror; goldtone crocodile skin pattern pop-up lip-view, maker unknown; centre American holder for lipstick and lipstick tissues, decorated with lips and a diamante eye, maker unknown.

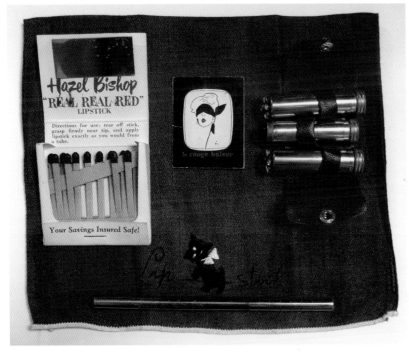

Hazel Bishop 'Real Real Red' Lipstick Matchbook; Rouge Baiser lipstick tissues; Revlon jewelled lipsticks in leather carrying case; Gala Lip Line; all resting on a scarlet lipstick handkerchief, 1950s.

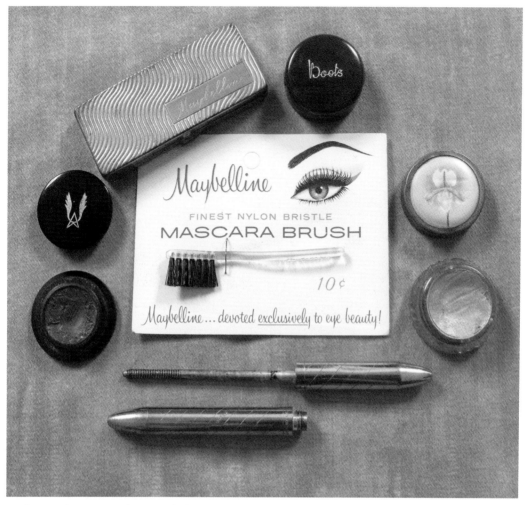

A collection of 1950s eye make-up. Maybelline mascara box and brush; Eye shadows left Elizabeth Arden; top Boots; right Leichner; and bottom, Helena Rubinstein's Mascaramatic, the first wand mascara.

bow that you covered with lipstick and pressed against your mouth. Movie make-up artist Ern Westmore designed 'Hollywood lip and eyebrow outlines'; pink plastic cut outs that could be placed over less than ideal lips and brows, and simply coloured in.

Eyes were another area of emphasis. Eyebrows were dark, thick and (hopefully) beautifully shaped. Eyelashes were curled and darkened. Helena Rubinstein's Mascaramatic, the first wand mascara, was launched in 1958 and provided a welcome alternative to the old-fashioned block mascara: 'Curls! Colours! Waterprooof Lashes! No water, no messy brush. Just opens like a pen.' Colourful eye shadows were recommended to coordinate with clothes and hair shade – typically blue for blondes, and green for brunettes. Film stars such as Audrey Hepburn popularised the exotic 'doe eyed look' (detractors called it 'Bride of Frankenstein') in which eyes were thickly lined with liquid kohl or pencil and swept into an almond shape; a style that reached its extravagant zenith in the following decade with Elizabeth Taylor's eye paint in the film *Cleopatra* (1963).

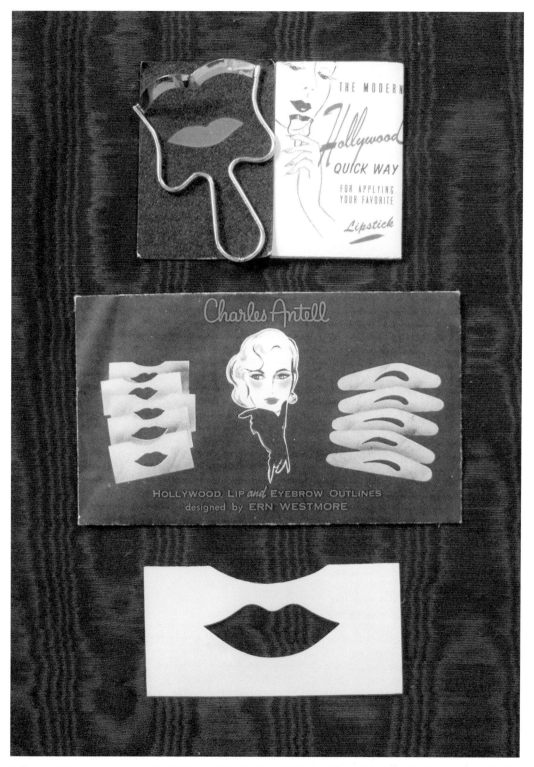

Hollywood 'Glamour Lips' applicator 1950s and Charles Antell Hollywod Lip and Eyebrow Outlines designed by Ern Westmore, 1940s/50s.

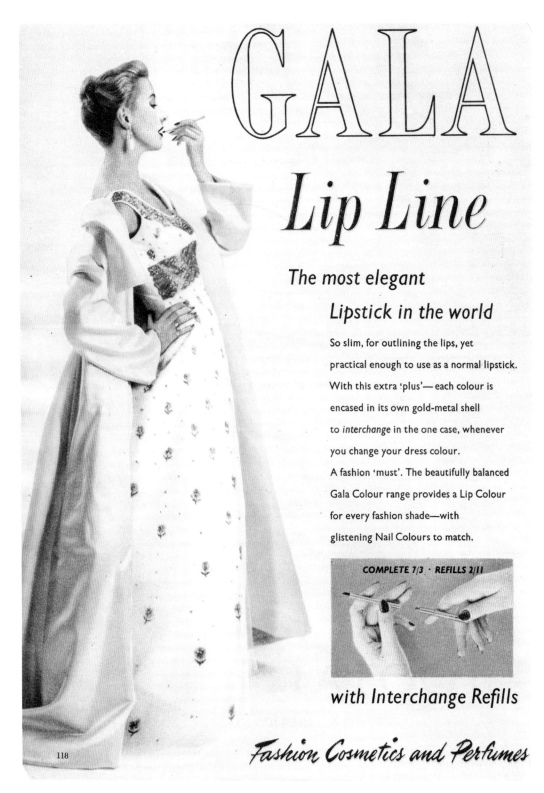

GALA
Lip Line

The most elegant
Lipstick in the world

So slim, for outlining the lips, yet
practical enough to use as a normal lipstick.
With this extra 'plus'— each colour is
encased in its own gold-metal shell
to *interchange* in the one case, whenever
you change your dress colour.
A fashion 'must'. The beautifully balanced
Gala Colour range provides a Lip Colour
for every fashion shade—with
glistening Nail Colours to match.

COMPLETE 7/3 · REFILLS 2/11

with Interchange Refills

Fashion Cosmetics and Perfumes

118

1948 Advertisement for Gala Lip Line.

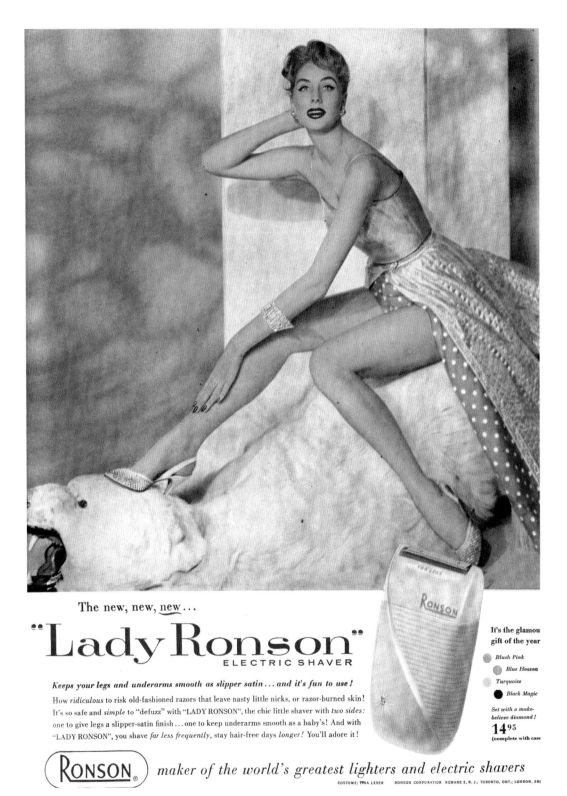

The new, new, new...

"Lady Ronson"
ELECTRIC SHAVER

It's the glamou
gift of the year

● Blush Pink
● Blue Heaven
○ Turquoise
● Black Magic

*Set with a make-
believe diamond!*

14⁹⁵
(complete with case

Keeps your legs and underarms smooth as slipper satin ... and it's fun to use!

How *ridiculous* to risk old-fashioned razors that leave nasty little nicks, or razor-burned skin!
It's so safe and *simple* to "defuzz" with "LADY RONSON", the chic little shaver with *two sides*:
one to give legs a slipper-satin finish ... one to keep underarms smooth as a baby's! And with
"LADY RONSON", you shave *far less frequently*, stay hair-free days *longer!* You'll adore it!

(RONSON.) *maker of the world's greatest lighters and electric shavers*

COSTUME: TINA LESER   RONSON CORPORATION NEWARE 2, N. J.; TORONTO, ONT.; LONDON, ENG

Lady Ronson electric shaver advertisement, 1956.

Perfect Grooming

Though the full on Queen of the Nile look was perhaps best reserved for parties, perfect grooming was expected at all times. Magazines suggested suitable 'maquillages' for every occasion, from going out on a first date to meeting your boyfriend's mother. 'Lesley didn't listen to the cynics who prescribed no make-up and a mousy act when she met prospective mum-in law,' advised a photo-story in *Woman* magazine in 1956. 'Her attractive yet unobtrusive make-up, her fresh perfect grooming and her charming naturalness are just the qualities that Gerry's mother always hoped to find in her son's future bride.'

'Perfect Grooming' (a favourite phrase of the decade) was stipulated from top to toe. 'The fashion for … gossamer stockings spotlights the perfection of legs and feet,' warned *Vogue* in 1954, recommending 'deep and cruel leg massage,' followed by a wax depilatory to make the skin 'as smooth as marble'. Foundation or pancake make-up was then to be applied to the legs to cover up any uneven colouring before carefully painting the toenails in graduated tones from crimson to palest pink. Marbled smoothness was facilitated by the introduction of the electric lady shave in the late forties, distinguished from male electric razors by pretty boudoir colours. 'Now – for the luxury of perfect grooming,' enticed a 1956 ad for the new Lady Ronson, which came in Blue Heaven or Blush Pink.

Strapless dresses made shaving the underarms a necessity and emphasised the importance of deodorant. Often supplied in cream form in a little tin or jar, deodorant underwent a revolution

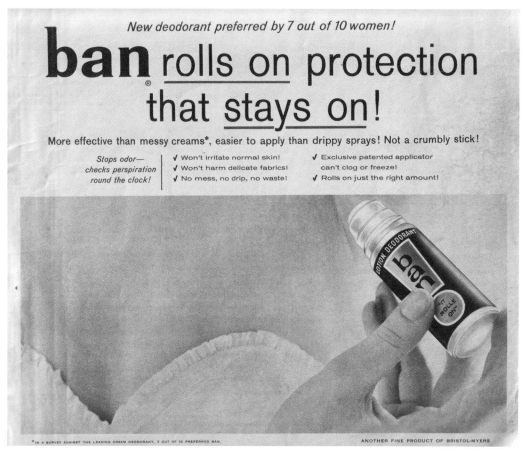

1950s advertisement for Ban Roll-On, the first roll-on deodorant.

in the early fifties. Helen Barnett Diserens worked for the Mum production team in the USA, and inspired by another new invention, Lazlo Biro's ballpoint pen, she came up with the first roll-on deodorant. Ban Roll-On launched in 1952 'less messy and easier to apply than creams' promised the ads.

Once you were hairless and odourless, you still had to be blemish free. Body make-up and powder applied to the décolletage created an unbroken line from the bust to the immaculately made up face. Ladies had no qualms about toucing up their make-up in public. Powder compacts and mirrored lip views were favourite fifties accessories, and came beautifully decorated in an endless variety of styles, designed to be displayed in company.

Coco Chanel, who reopened her Paris Fashion House in 1954, was deeply unimpressed both by strapless evening dresses 'Nothing is uglier for a woman; boned horrors, that's what they are,' and by ladies powdering their noses during meals and placing their gilded vanity cases on the table. 'How can one be elegant doing that?' she demanded grumpily. 'And all those women who leave lipstick all over table napkins and on glasses. I tell them, when you come to my house I will provide you with paper napkins, my table linen is too fine to be spoilt by you.'

Designer Luxury
Chanel was however in a minority. Fashion houses were increasingly coming to realise that perfumes and cosmetics were a major way of promoting their name and raising their turnover by providing a bit of designer luxury for the thousands of women who could never hope to afford a piece of original couture. Christian Dior launched a cosmetics line in 1956 including a lipstick that had a silver and gold case for the handbag, and a luxurious Baccarat crystal container – modelled on the obelisk in the place de la Concorde – for display on the dressing table.

Chanel's great rival Schiaparelli designed nail varnish colours for Cutex as well as selling her own famous series of perfumes, powders and lipsticks in their distinctive shocking pink boxes.

Cosmetic advertising and packaging attracted some of the most remarkable artists of the day. Salvador Dali produced perfume bottle designs for Schiaparelli and in 1950 Elgin American commissioned him to create a powder compact in the shape of a bird with folded wings: 'A Dali Flight of Fancy … exultant expression of an artist's dream … lofty spirit of fashion released from all earthbound tradition,' enthused the advertisement. Some contemporaries criticised Salvador Dali for his profitable involvement in fashion and commerce. André Breton, founding member of the Surrealist movement, nicknamed him Avida Dollars (anag.) – but today Dali's *Bird-in-Hand* is one of the rarest and most desirable of all vanity cases.

As well as being beautifully presented, make-up itself became increasingly luxurious – filled with exotic ingredients ranging from royal jelly to turtle oil to caviar. Helena Rubinstein created lipstick and foundation from 'Pure Atomised silk'; Lily Daché produced a face powder made from crushed pearls; Placentubex 'the newest skin food of all' promised to remove wrinkles with the help of an entirely natural ingredient, placenta. Prices could be equally extravagant.

Estée Lauder, who started her skincare business in New York in 1946, aimed straight for the top end of the market. Her first US Department store account was with Saks Fifth Avenue, and her international debut was with Harrods. Though she pioneered free samples (today an accepted part of cosmetics marketing) the whole point of these 'free' gifts was to encourage women to spend as much as possible on costly face products. In 1958 Lauder launched her famous Re-Nutritive Cream, priced at an astonishing $115, and said to be the most expensive cream in the world.

The Age of Boom
Post-war desire for pleasure and prettiness had created an unparalleled market for cosmetics. By 1957 women in the USA were spending around 4 billion dollars a year on make-up and skin care

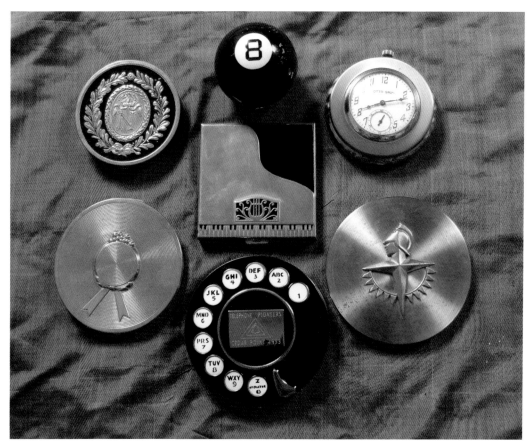

A collection of powder compacts. Clockwise from top – American '8 Ball' compact (unmarked) 1940s/50s; Watch compact by Otto Grun 1950s; 1951 Festival of Britain compact by Le Rage; American Telephone Dial compact, dated 1953 (unmarked); Picture Hat compact by Dorothy Gray 1940s; Elizabeth Arden Napolenic compact. 1954; Piano compact by Volupté, USA 1950s.

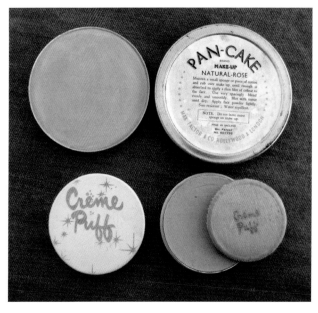

Max Factor Pan-Cake make-up and Creme Puff, 1950s.

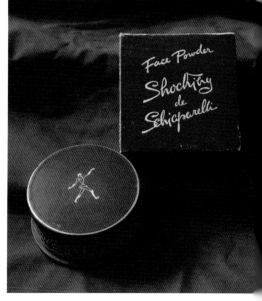

Schiaparelli Shocking powder box, c.1950s.

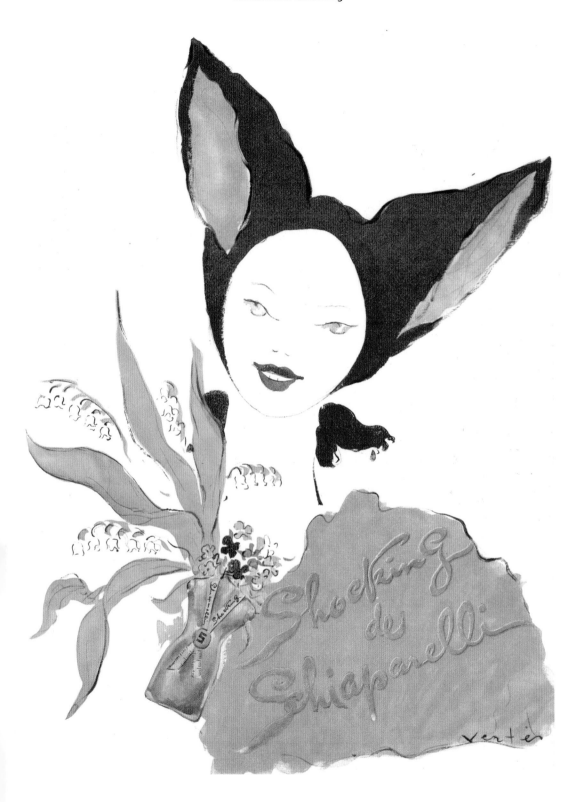

1940s advertisement for Schiaparelli's Shocking perfume designed by Marcel Vertes.

and even Britain had shrugged off the last vestiges of rationing and was happily embracing the squander bug. 'When did you last hear the word austerity?' demanded *Queen* magazine in their famous 'Boom' issue of Sept 1959. 'At this minute there is more money in Britain than ever before. Britain has launched into an era of unparalleled lavish living … You are living in a new world; you are living in a boom.'

Along with the champagne, the Rolls-Royces, and the modern penthouse flats filled with televisions and electronic typewriters, the development of the beauty business epitomised this age of boom. *Queen* highlighted the popularity of cosmetic surgery, the emergence of super-luxury brands (Elizabeth Arden's face creams; Jean Patou's Joy perfume) and the rise of rampant consumerism. 'There is a new philosophy in accessory buying – simply, buying more. Where women used to buy one …"to go with everything", they now buy a lipstick to go with each dress or suit,' observed the magazine under a photograph of twenty-two must-have modern lipsticks.

Travel
Travelling for pleasure (impossible during the war years), was another preoccupation of this boom generation at every level of the market from Butlin's holiday camps to flights abroad.

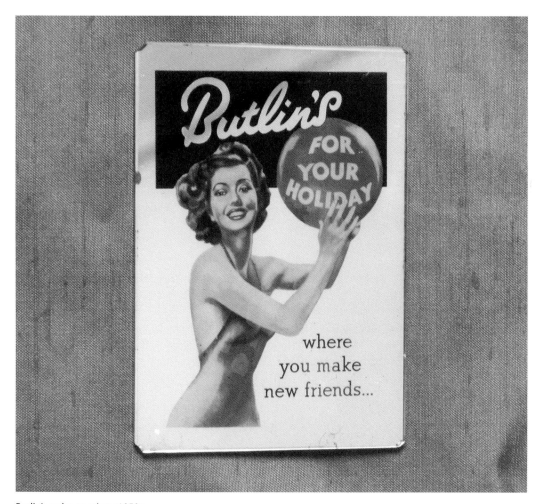

Butlin's make-up mirror, 1950s.

The world's first airport duty-free shop opened at Shannon airport in Ireland in 1947 and, as the Twentieth Century progressed, buying cosmetics and fragrances at the airport gradually became an essential part of the holiday experience. BOAC launched the world's first tourist airfares in 1952 (presaging the package holiday) and the immaculately made-up air hostess – her perfect grooming reflecting both the sexiness and safety of air travel – became one of the icons of the age, and a career role model for little girls. In the following decade both Barbie and Sindy – reliable indicators of female aspirations – were given air hostess' uniforms.

Travel was also a major decorative theme. Powder compacts, shaped like suitcases and emblazoned with miniature luggage labels, were produced for airlines and cruise ships. Souvenir compacts recorded tourist sights from the Empire State Building to Piccadilly Circus. Even if you never got any closer to France than a sniff of French perfume, Parisian scenes – featuring cafes, ladies in New Look frocks – and the French poodle, were popular fifties images, appearing not just on cosmetic items but across fashion and the decorative arts.

Travel also had a major impact on the health and beauty industry. With the growth in foreign holidays and arrival of the bikini (named after Bikini Atoll, site of nuclear weapons tests in 1946) sales of suntan products boomed.

Many famous brands had been developed in the late 1930s. The founder of L'Oréal, chemist Eugene Schueller, created Ambre Solaire in 1936. Two years later Franz Greiter, a young chemistry student (who was badly sunburnt whilst climbing Piz Buin mountain in Austria), set up a small laboratory in his parent's home and devised a new protective product, Gletscher Crème (Glacier Cream), the foundation for the Piz Buin company.

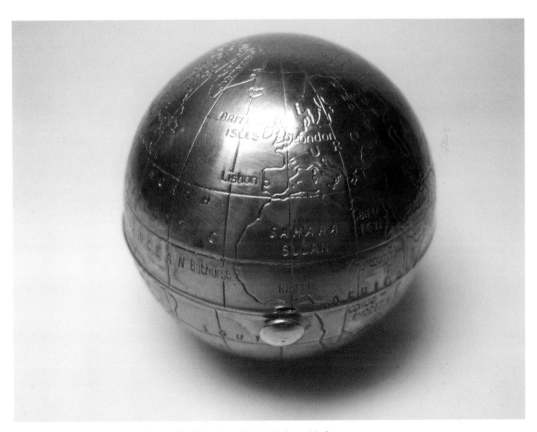

Compact by Pygmalion in the shape of a globe, 1951. *Gray's Antiques Market*

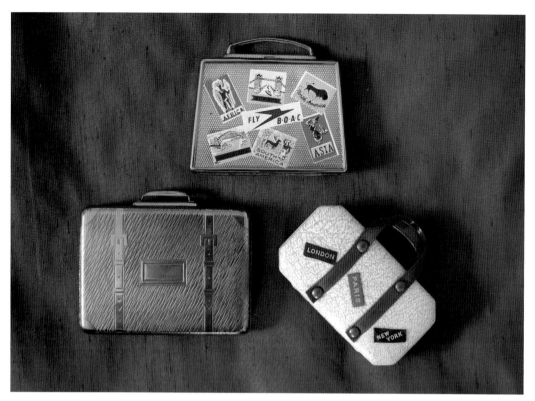

1950s Travel compacts: goldtone suitcase by Kigu – inner lid inscribed Bon Voyage; BOAC goldtone handbag compact decorated with luggage labels by Mascot (trade name of British firm A.S. Brown); vinyl, metal and plastic miniature manicure set in the form of a suitcase with labels.

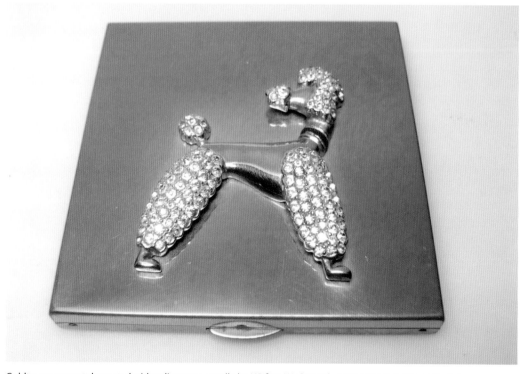

Goldtone compact decorated with a diamante poodle by US firm Wadsworth, 1950s. *Gray's Antiques Market*

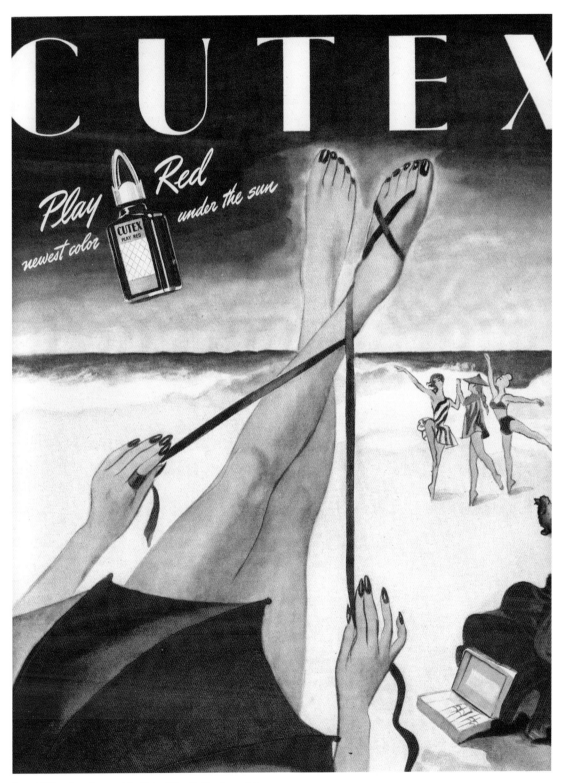

Late 1940s advertisement for Cutex 'Play Red' nail varnish.

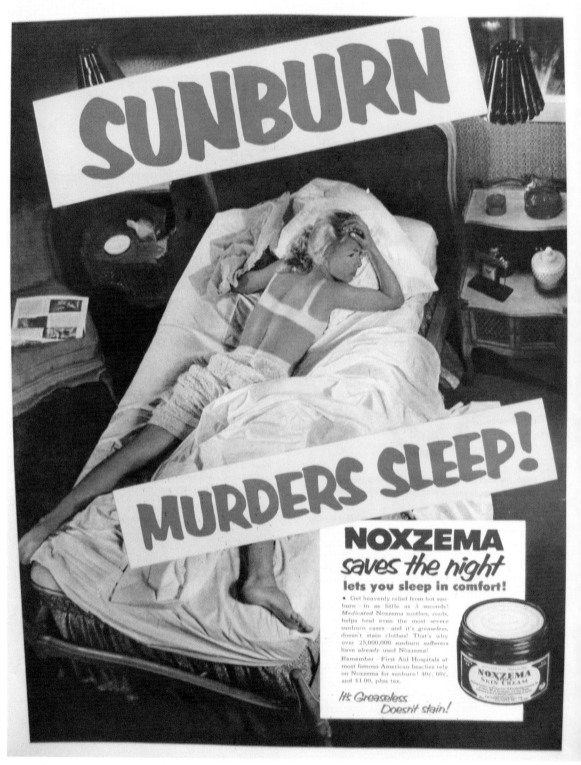

1950s advertisement for Noxzema Sunburn Relief Skin cream.

Whilst WWII interrupted both holidays and the commercial sales of tanning lotions, sunscreens were important for military use. In 1944 Florida pharmacist and airman Benjamin Green developed 'Red Vet Pet' in his kitchen. Similar to petroleum jelly, the cream that was designed to protect soldiers from ultra violet radiation and provided the basis for the best-selling Coppertone Suntan Cream. World War II also promoted the development of another holiday essential. Ray Ban (est.1937) supplied anti-glare aviator glasses for US army and navy pilots. After the war Ray-Ban's Wayfarers (designed in 1952) became arguably the most famous sunglasses in the world. They were worn by everyone from James Dean to Marilyn Monroe to Audrey Hepburn, and a pair of shades became one of the accessories of stardom.

Even with dark glasses to cover your eyes, full make-up was still recommended for the beach. *Vogue*'s summer, sand and sea essentials for 1954 included Max Factor's 'Sun Frolic' Creme Puff; two types of powder light and dark, to go with your suntan, housed in Elizabeth Arden's elegant Napoleonic-style compacts; and a range of lipsticks, nail varnish and eye shadows to match bathing suits and sundresses.

Ding Dong – Avon Calling

With make-up being worn everywhere, even on the beach, it was a boom time for cosmetics manufacturers too, and none more so than Avon.

The US firm was founded in 1886. David McConnell, a travelling bible salesman, decided to offer a little bottle of perfume as an incentive with each purchase. When he discovered that the scent was more popular than the good book, he established The California Perfume Company, recruiting women to sell door-to-door. In 1939 the firm's name was changed to Avon (inspired by McConnell's love of Shakespeare) and after the war, as demand for luxury products grew, so did Avon. By the mid-fifties the company was producing over 500 different beauty products and had an annual turnover of $55 million. The post-war generation of housewives provided an enthusiastic audience and a massive potential workforce. Women seeking work that would not interfere with family life were seduced by the chance of making some pin money, by the attraction of female companionship, and by brilliant advertising. The phrase 'Ding, Dong, Avon Calling' first featured on a TV commercial in 1954. It became one of the most famous slogans of the day and the 'immaculately groomed' Avon lady, with her kit of creams and cosmetics, was like the air hostess, another smartly dressed icon of the decade.

Grown-up Glamour

On the one hand the predominant female look of the 1950s was distinctly grown-up: whether it was the womanly curves of Marilyn Monroe; the perfectly made-up Avon lady; or the poised elegance of famous fashion models of the decade – Barbara Goalen, Fiona Campbell-Walter, Bronwen Pugh – aloof thoroughbreds who, if they weren't members of the aristocracy already, looked as though they would undoubtedly marry into it (and mostly did).

Hat, gloves, a smart suit, matching shoes and handbag were the accepted outfit for a woman going into town, and the gilded powder compact – a favourite gift for girls approaching adulthood – ensured ladylike perfection at all times.

But by the end of the decade change was in the air. Audrey Hepburn, though matchlessly elegant, had a gamine quality that epitomised the modern age and anticipated the youthful styles of the sixties. 'Nobody ever looked like her before World War II,' observed Cecil Beaton. 'She wears no powder, so that her white skin has a bright sheen. Using a stick of greasepaint with a deft stroke she liberally smudges both upper and lower eyelids with black … Audrey Hepburn is the gamine, the urchin, the lost Barnardo Boy … She is a wistful child of a war chided era.'

The children of the war had grown up into a new phenomenon: 'Teenagers' who, thanks to post-war employment, had become an increasingly powerful and independent force. They didn't

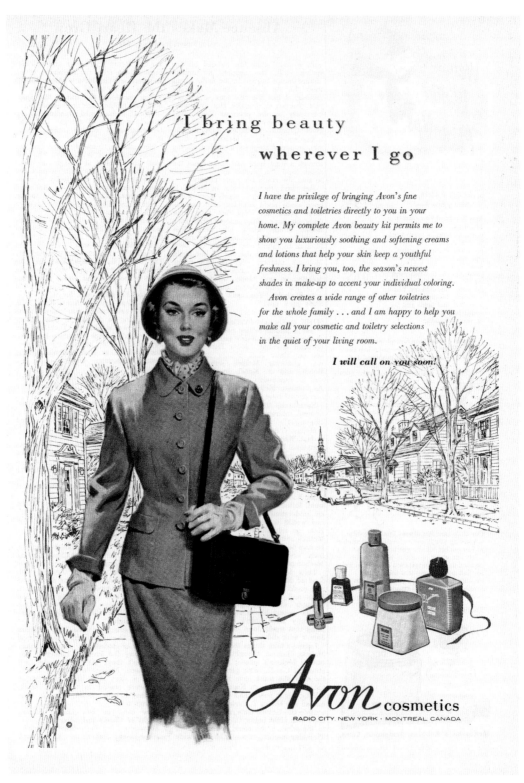

I bring beauty
wherever I go

I have the privilege of bringing Avon's fine
cosmetics and toiletries directly to you in your
home. My complete Avon beauty kit permits me to
show you luxuriously soothing and softening creams
and lotions that help your skin keep a youthful
freshness. I bring you, too, the season's newest
shades in make-up to accent your individual coloring.

Avon creates a wide range of other toiletries
for the whole family . . . and I am happy to help you
make all your cosmetic and toiletry selections
in the quiet of your living room.

I will call on you soon!

Avon cosmetics
RADIO CITY, NEW YORK · MONTREAL, CANADA

1950s Avon Advertisement.

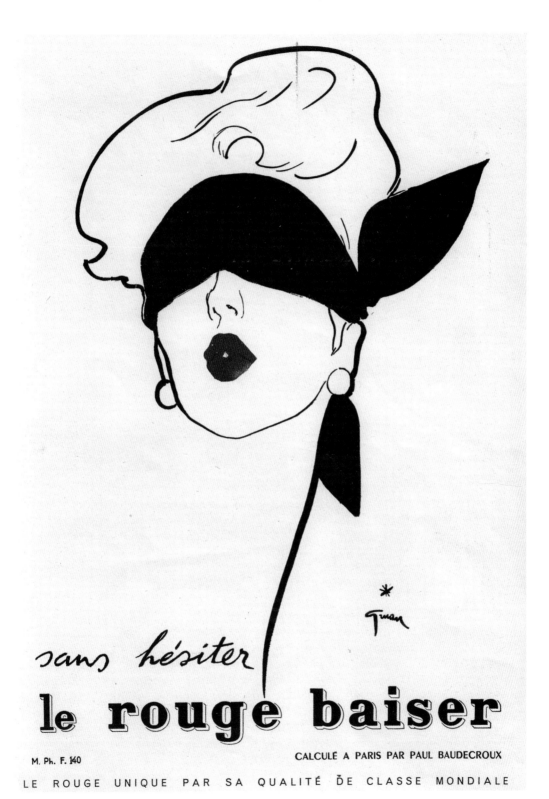

1949 advertisement for Rouge Baiser *La femme au Bandeau*, by artist René Gruau.

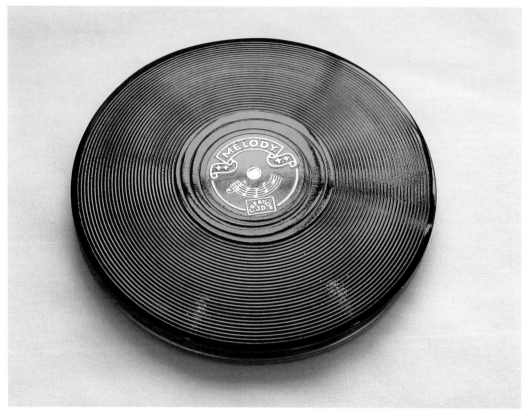

Melody powder compact in the form of a black vinyl record, 1950s.

want to dress or be like their parents and, with money in their pocket, they didn't have to. They had their own clubs and coffee bars; their own fashions inspired by street style and American films; and their own music – jazz, and rock and roll. A new breed of denim-clad rebel heroes from James Dean to Elvis Presley expressed their alienation from the adult world. 'What're you rebelling against, Johnny?' 'Whaddya got?' replied Marlon Brando in *The Wild One*. The fifties saw the beginning of the teenage revolution that was to define the 1960s – changing ideals of beauty and make-up along with everything else.

On The Post-War Dressing Table
The post-war period was a golden age not just for the creation of new beauty products but for the decoration of cosmetic containers and accessories.

The powder compact epitomised the period desire for fun and frivolity. In 1946 the New York firm Volupté launched their Golden Gesture compact in the shape of a hand, which appeared in various forms; plain, with jewellery, and even wearing a 'gay nineties' lace mitten. Four years later, as part of a series of 'Collector's Items', Volupté introduced the Petit Boudoir, a compact inspired by Marie Antoinette's dressing table, and which came with folding legs so that it could stand on display or be carried in a handbag. Not to be outdone rival US firm Wadsworth brought out a similar model, inspired by a French Eighteenth Century vanity table.

American companies came up with innumerable novelty shapes and compacts were modelled in the form of everything from telephone dials to pool balls, often found in a somewhat battered condition today, because of a sphere's natural tendency to roll off the table.

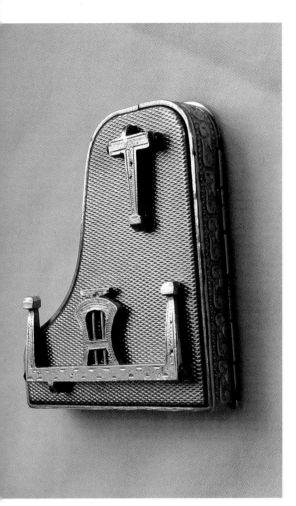

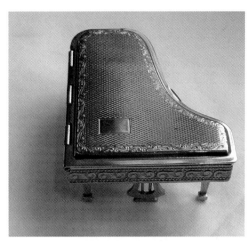

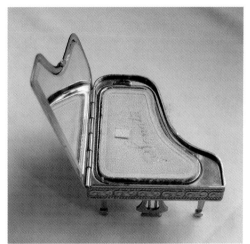

Sonato Piano compact by Pygmalion, with folding legs, 1950s.

Petite Boudoir compact by Volupté, c.1950. *Gray's Antiques Market*

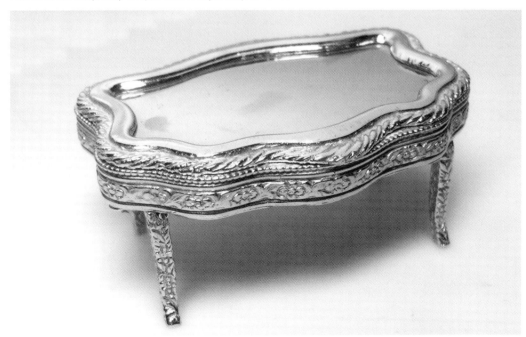

Once austerity restrictions were finally lifted, British firms too created innovative designs. Stratton resumed production in 1946 and two years later devised a compact with a self-opening inner lid – designed to make it easier to open without breaking the finger nails – and identified by a distinctive 'Compact-in-Hand' trademark, which remained in use till c.1970.

Kigu, established in London in 1947 by Hungarian émigré and third generation jeweller George Kiashek, devised a famous compact in the form of a flying saucer reflecting post-war fascination with space travel. Pygmalion created vanity cases shaped like globes and grand pianos.

Music and dance were favourite subjects. Ballet dancers appeared on many vanity cases and a classic example of fifties' kitsch was the musical manicure set or jewellery box, that opened up to reveal a plastic ballerina, pirouetting in front of a mirror, a perfect accessory for the kidney shaped, ruffled dressing table – fifties' furnishing at its most feminine.

Twinkling with diamante, decorated with flowers and romantic scenes, on the one hand compacts and cosmetic accessories were the ultimate 'girlie' items; but they also expressed more adult pleasures. Smoking, drinking and gambling were popular decorative images and a new fifties' fashion was the miniature ashtray compact, which could be slipped inside a handbag.

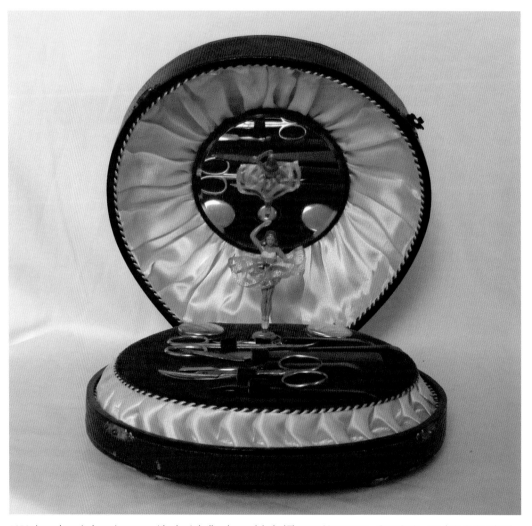

1950s boxed musical manicure set with plastic ballet dancer, labeled Thorens Movement – Ganz Paris – made in Switzerland.

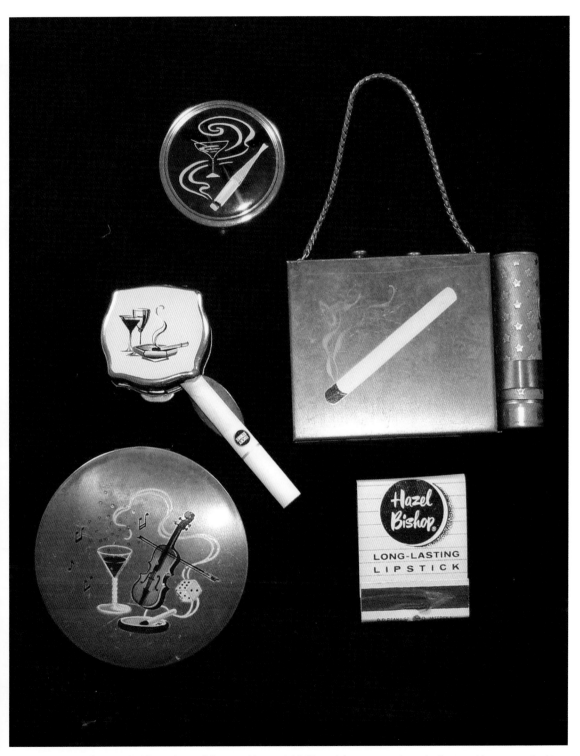

Stratton compact decorated with music, gambling, smoking and drinking; pink compact ashtray by Stratton; blue compact ashtray by Kigu; American chained vanity/cigarette case decorated with a cigarette. A book of real matches advertising Hazel Bishop Long Lasting Lipstick, 1950s.

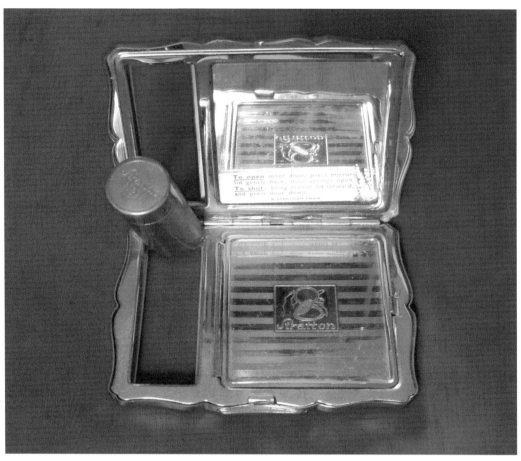

Stratton compact (open and closed) with pop-up lipstick – inner liner showing the Compact-in-Hand trademark, 1950s.

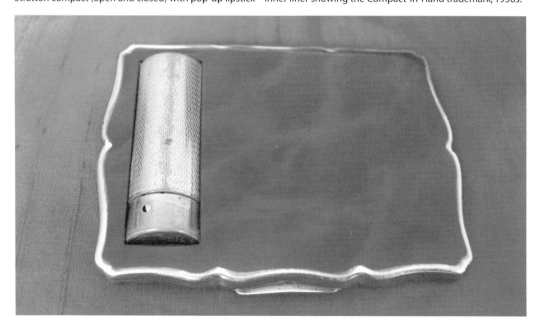

Many different designs were produced for lipsticks, lip-brushes and mirrored lip views. Revlon produced a leather-bound set of three lipstick cases decorated with rhinestones; a miniature plastic whiskey bottle opened to reveal a scarlet lipstick; a needlework purse came with compartments for lipstick, lip blotters and a mirror in the shape of a pair of lips. Scarlet handkerchiefs, so that you could blot your lipstick without leaving a visible stain, were another favourite handbag accessory. Mascara boxes came with integral mirrors and with the introduction of the wand mascara Stratton even produced a mirrored 'eye-view' that could be slipped over a mascara or eye pencil.

In one sense new materials and technology developed during WWII enhanced compacts and cosmetic packaging. Manufacturing processes were refined; improvements in materials and injection moulding resulted in plastics that were more affordable and less brittle than their pre-war equivalents. New materials such as Acrylic (aka Lucite and Perspex) became popular for vanity items; and plastic was used to provide easy to clean inner-liners, and imaginative exteriors.

The Trio-ette 'a fashion miracle of moulded tenite', made by the New York company Platé in 1946, was an elaborate triple compact (containing powder, rouge and lipstick) modelled on a Victorian hand mirror and costing only $5.50. With the development of mass production however, cheap and disposable plastic containers would eventually dominate cosmetic packaging and if the fifties was a golden age for the imaginative powder compact, it was also its apogee.

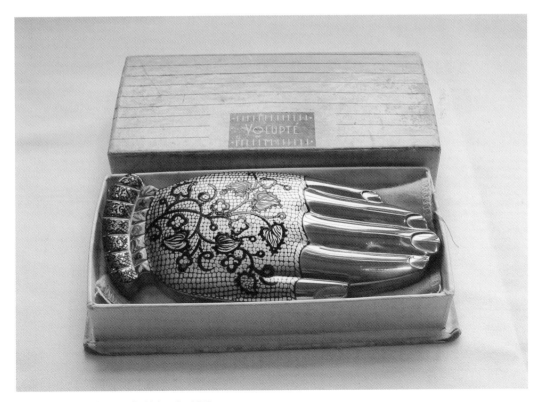

Gay Nineties Mitt Compact by Volupté, c.1948.

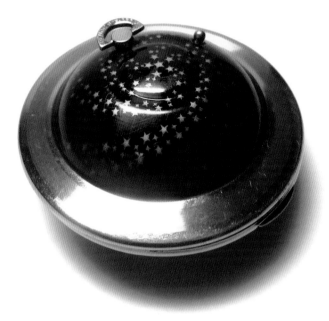

Kigu Flying Saucer compact, 1950s. Capturing period fascination with space travel, the musical version of this famous compact is very sought after by collectors. *Grays Antiques.*

Ballet compact, 1950s. Maker unknown. *Grays Antiques.*

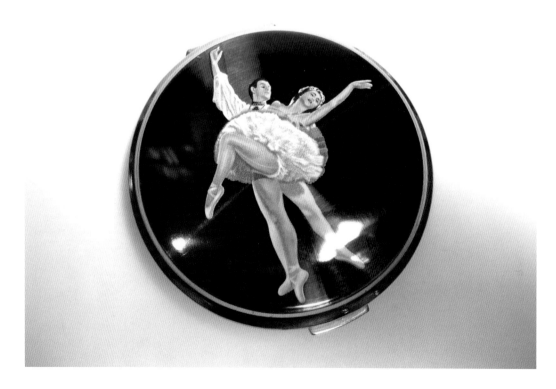

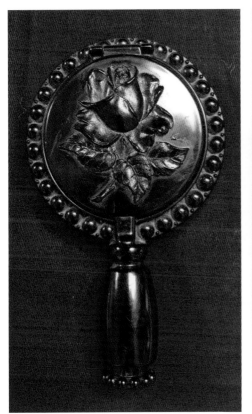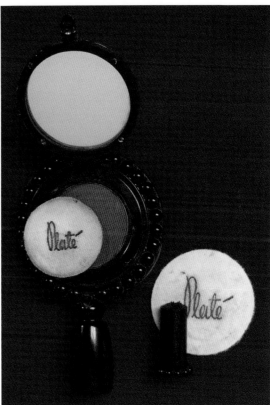

Trio-ette plastic vanity mirror compact by Platé, late 1940s.

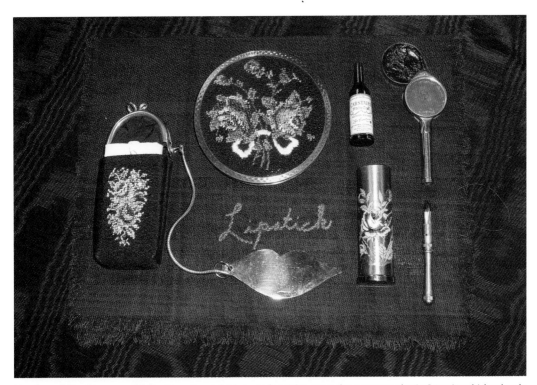

Needlework lipstick purse with lip-shaped metal mirror and matching powder compact; plastic Carstairs whiskey bottle concealing miniature red lipstick; lipstick mirror, with a swing out lipstick compartment and pull-out brush in the handle; rose decorated goldtone lipstick tube. All resting on a red lipstick handkerchief, 1950s.

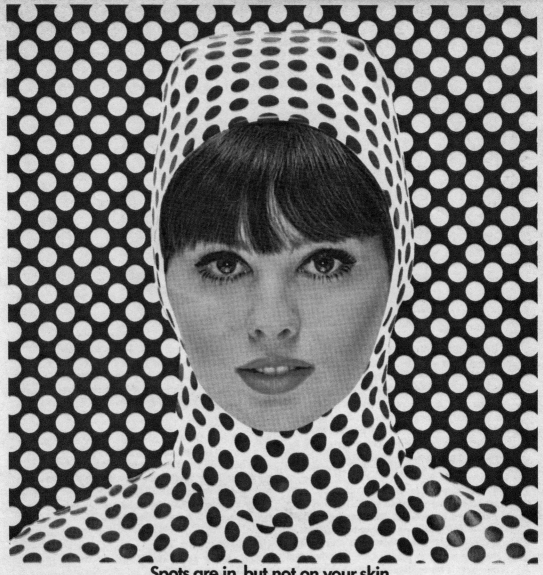

Spots are in, but not on your skin

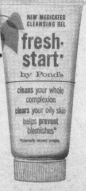

NEW MEDICATED CLEANSING GEL

fresh-start
by Pond's

cleans your whole complexion
clears your oily skin
helps prevent blemishes*

*Externally caused pimples

New Fresh-Start® by Pond's cleans out oil-choked pore openings, the breeding ground for blemishes*

Who wants a spotty, polka-dotty skin? If up to now you haven't been able to get rid of those spots, here's a cleanser that cuts the breeding ground right out from under them! Fresh-Start is a marvelous new greaseless gel that cleans out the dirt . . . clears away the oil that can cause blemishes . . . tingles, tones, medicates your skin till it *sparkles!* Wash with icy-fresh, tingling Fresh-Start twice a day to help prevent blemishes. Wear between cleansings to protect and medicate invisibly. It's the new unbeatable way to help you look sparkling—and *spotless!*

*Externally caused pimples

Advertisement for Fresh-Start by Pond's, 1966.

CHAPTER NINE

Swinging Make-up
Beauty in the 1960s

THROUGHOUT THE history of fashion curves tend to be followed by straight lines. If the ideal of the fifties was the hourglass silhouette epitomised by Jayne Mansfield with her fabulous 44 inch bust then the shape of the sixties was very different. Lesley Hornby was 5ft 6, weighed just under six and a half stone and had a bust measurement of 30½ inches. Her slender figure inspired the nickname which was to become famous across the world. 'This is the Face of 1966,' declared the *Daily Express* in 1966. 'Twiggy, The Cockney Kid with a face to launch a thousand shapes ... And she's only 16.'

So this was the New Look of the sixties; straight up and down, skinny, leggy, and above all breathtakingly young.

'You're sixteen, you're beautiful and you're mine!'

The most important influence on sixties fashion and make-up is that this was the age of the teenager. The baby boomers had matured into adolescents and in a booming economy they had money or 'bread' in the fashionable slang of the day. By 1965 fifty per cent of all the clothes produced in Britain were being bought by kids aged 15-19: in America, that same year teenagers spent $3.5billion on clothes.

Because youth had the spending power, fashion changed accordingly. Swinging London took over from couture Paris as the epicentre of style and the boutique replaced the traditional department store. The latest looks developed from the street upwards and, perhaps for the first time, girls no longer wanted to look like their mothers, it was their mothers who wanted to look like them. 'Suddenly every girl with a hope of getting away with it is aiming to look not only under voting age, but under the age of consent,' declared Mary Quant, who from her boutique in London's King's Road observed the Chelsea girls, and pioneered the fashions that made London swing; the plastic mac, kinky boots, the trouser suit and most famously the miniskirt.

In 1967 *The Guardian* asked Mary Quant what was the focus of modern day fashion and she answered quite simply 'the crutch'. Bend over too quickly in a miniskirt and you were in danger of revealing it, hence stockings and suspenders being replaced by tights (another Mary Quant innovation). The miniskirt was blamed for everything from the moral decline of the nation's youth to an increase in traffic accidents as drivers took their eyes off the road. Everyone from Quant to Courrèges claimed responsibility for inventing the mini, but it was certainly the girls of swinging

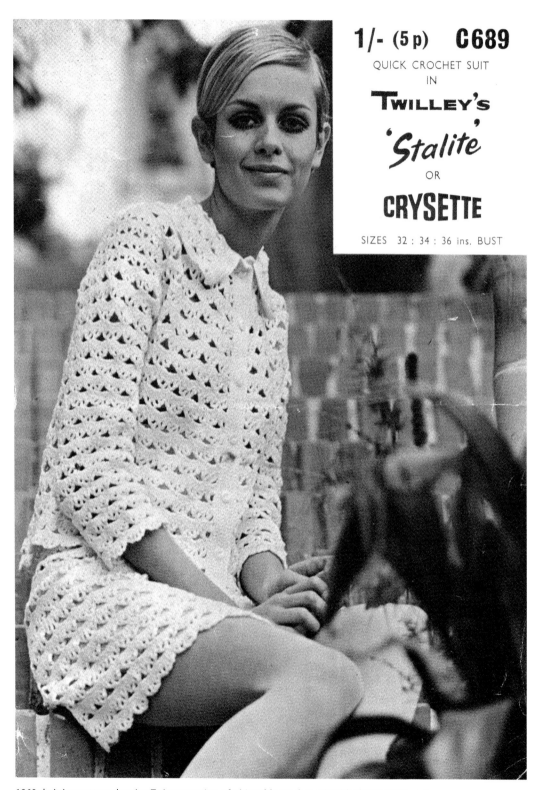

1/- (5p) **C689**
QUICK CROCHET SUIT
IN
TWILLEY'S
'*Stalite*'
OR
CRYSETTE

SIZES 32 : 34 : 36 ins. BUST

1960s knitting pattern showing Twiggy wearing a fashionable crochet suit with classic 1960s make-up.

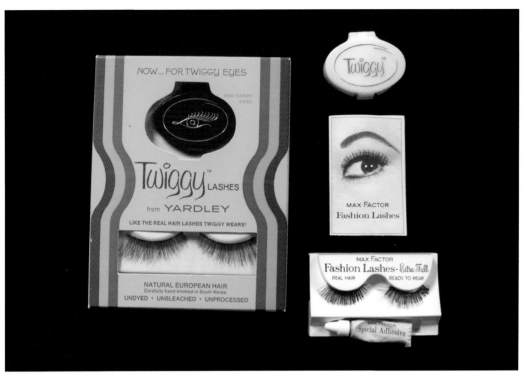

Twiggy Lashes by Yardley made from 'natural European hair', c.1967; Twiggy eye shadow by Yardley (black and white), c.1967; Max Factor Fashion Lashes. 1960s.

Avon lipsticks, late 1960s.

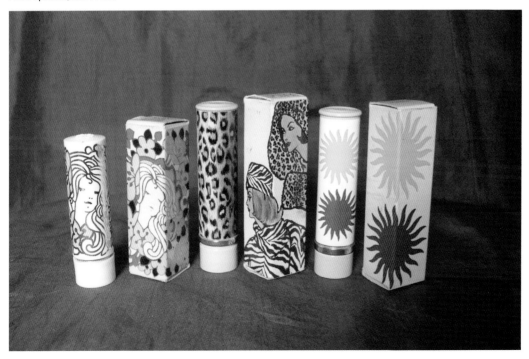

1960s make-up mirror from Just Looking – a fashionable London boutique.

London who made the skirt famous across the world. When Mary Quant took a posse of London models to America, the mini took the US by storm. 'The miniskirt will enable girls to run faster, and because of it, they may have to,' warned the Mayor of New York; but in one sense running was what the sixties were all about.

The ladylike fifties stiletto was cast off in favour of the round-toed, little girlish Mary Jane and the low-heeled fashion boot, perfect for go-go dancing in one of the new 'discothèques'. Rather than being photographed in elegantly static poses, the latest young models (Twiggy, Jean 'the Shrimp' Shrimpton, Penelope Tree) were captured by a new generation of trendy working-class photographers (David Bailey, Terrence Donovan) running, jumping, dancing and rejoicing in their youth.

Swinging Make-up

Cosmetics reflected this new youthful ideal, and were essential for obtaining it. 'What a great many people still don't realise is that the Look isn't just the garments you wear,' wrote Mary Quant in her autobiography in 1966. 'It's the way you put the make-up on, the way you do your hair … even the way you smoke your fag. All these are part of the same 'feeling'. Make-up – old style – is out. It is used as expertly as ever but it is not designed to show. The ideal now is to look as though you have a baby skin untouched by cosmetics.'

The heavy pancake of the fifties was replaced by a new range of lighter more youthful foundations and the cosmetic buzzwords of the decade were 'translucent', 'natural' and 'light': Ultra Lucent by Max Factor, 'Ultra light! Ultra sheen! Ultra Natural!'; Estée Lauder's See Through Make-up, 'Let your own Natural Beauty Shine through'; Helena Rubinstein's Cover Fluid, 'Gossamer light, soft translucent glow. Natural Beauty'. Mary Quant was typically cheeky with her 'Starkers Nude Foundation', part of the Quant cosmetics range launched in 1966 and which promised 'the bare essentials for the bare look'.

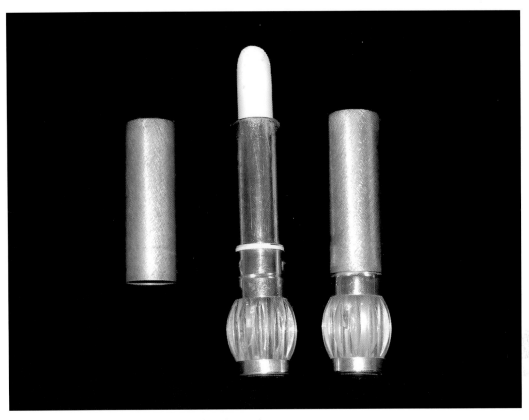

White lipstick – gilt metal and Perspex swivel base by Vanda, 1960s.

Pale lips replaced the sensual, sticky scarlets of the previous decade. White lipstick was a favourite with young Mods (short for Modernist) and see-through pink glosses were a best-seller. Manufacturers added titanium to make lipstick iridescent. Shiny metallic cosmetics complemented the space-age fashions created by Paris designers Pierre Cardin, André Courrèges and Paco Rabanne who sent their models down the catwalk in chain mail dresses and silver trousers. Helena Rubinstein launched lipsticks called 'Bronze Rage! Silver Rage! Gold Rage!' and Revlon's Moon Drops lipstick created a wet-look pearly sheen. Lipsticks might have been pale, but their packaging became increasingly decorative, seducing young purchasers with sweetshop colours and trendy images.

With lips being muted, the main emphasis was on the eyes. 'There you can use the lot,' advised Quant, 'eye shadow, eyeliner and lashings of mascara plus false eyelashes – even false eyebrows I should think – provided you've managed to master the art of putting them on and keeping them in place.'

Elizabeth Taylor created a vogue for Cleopatra eyes: bright eye shadow emphasised by thick lines of pencil or liquid liner; a dramatic look that that required a very steady hand and non-running make-up to avoid resembling a panda.

False eyelashes could be equally challenging. Jean Shrimpton remembered that if you weren't careful you could end up with 'a nasty, gummy line of white glue showing on the eyelid, which was torture to get off'. False eyelashes could come loose, landing on your dress like furry caterpillars or worst of all, remembers one magazine editor, 'if you wore them on the upper and the lower lashes they had an unfortunate tendency to lock together.'

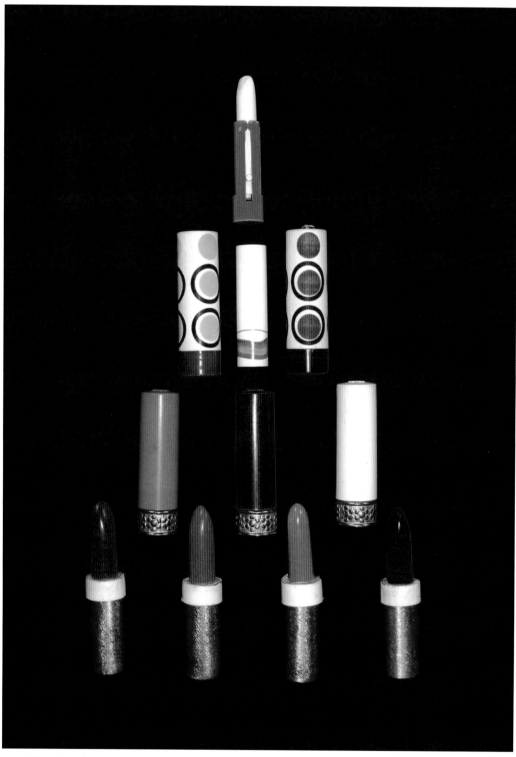

1960s Plastic lipsticks: white lipstick unmarked; lipsticks decorated with day glow circles by Yardley; plastic and gilt base lipsticks by Avon; Max Factor lipstick testers.

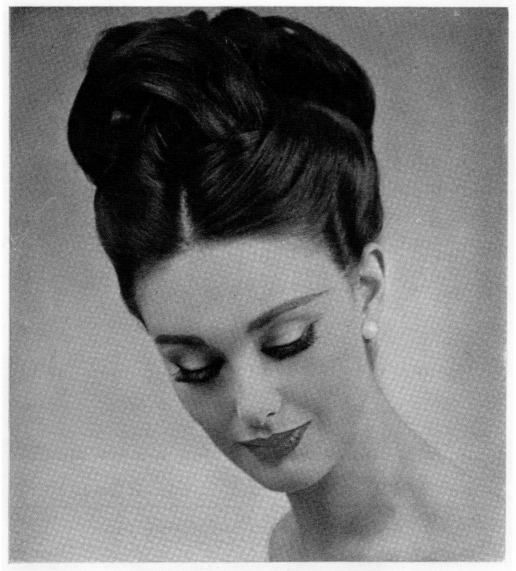

THE MONTEIL LOOK

. . . is one of serene poise, born of utter confidence in your own beauty. Shown here, the ingredients:
—for your skin, Monteil's new "Color-Blend," a pastel complexion-maker applied with an artist's brush
—for the beautifully "sculptured" eye, "Platinum" and "Taupe" Eye Shadows and a "Navy Blue" Eye Liner
—and for your lips, "Cherry Brandy" Super-Lumium Lipstick, one of Monteil's bright new "Vintage" shades.
Put them together and see how *you* look in "The Monteil Look."

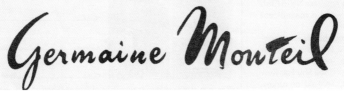

Advertisement for Germaine Monteil cosmetics, 1963, showing a beehive hairdo.

175

'False eyelashes now come in about 40 types', observed *Vogue* in 1966 and the point of all this decoration, was to increase the big-eyed, baby look, most famously displayed by Twiggy. She would take half an hour or more just to do her eyes, applying three sets of false eyelashes to her upper lids, and using a fine brush to paint lower lashes, underneath the eye, a look inspired by a doll. Young girls imitated her, drawing 'Twiggies' underneath their eyes and in the US Yardley brought out 'Twiggystix' eye pencils and Twiggy eye shadows and lashes. So an apparently 'natural' complexion was countered by rampant artificiality, and not just when it came to stick-on eyelashes.

Beehives, Wigs and Bobs

The late fifties and the first half of the sixties saw the fashion for the towering beehive hairdo – also known as the B-52, after the bulbous nose of the B-52 bomber. Hair was wound round rollers; dried under a hooded drier; backcombed to achieve the maximum bouffant effect; before being fixed with lashings of aerosol hairspray. Britain's first TV hairdresser, Raymond of Mayfair, became known as Mr Teasy Weasy because of his elaborate teased styles, accessorised with ornaments and extra hairpieces.

By the mid-sixties wigs were the literal height of fashion. They came in every style and enabled a girl to completely change her look. In 1966 the *Daily Express* recommended the 'Smoochy', a fashionable silver grey wig that covered half of the face 'specially designed for the not so pretty

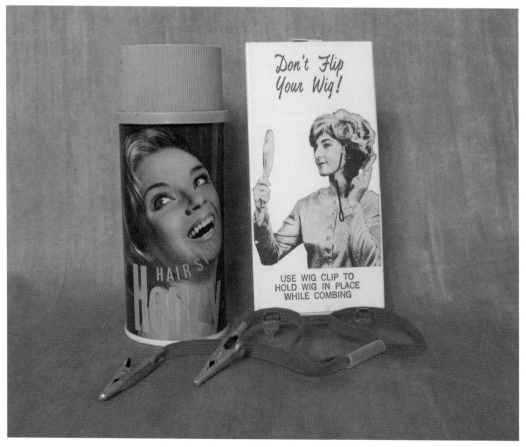

Richard Henry Hairspray and Don't Flip Your Wig wig clip, 1960s.

girl'. According to London's top hairdressers, seventy-five per cent of customers had at least one if not several wigs. 'Many girls are having their hair chopped off, but within two weeks they are back asking for a long hairpiece,' Arthur of Baker Street (London's busiest wig salon) told *Vogue*, and demand for wigs was stimulated by the short geometric haircuts, that were an essential part of the sixties look.

In the sixties, British teenagers shook up hairstyles as well as fashion. The Beatles' mop-tops were copied across the world and Twiggy shot to fame after her fragile beauty was revealed by a boyish crop from Leonard of Mayfair. Mary Quant and her models popularised the new geometric styles developed by London crimper Vidal Sassoon; creator of the Bob, the Five Point Cut, and Mia Farrow's Urchin cut, designed for her role in *Rosemary's Baby* in 1968. British hairstyles became famous across the world and hairdressers, previously anonymous figures providing a discreet service to their clients, became part of the new popocracy and celebrities in their own right.

By 1968, British teenagers were spending £13 million a year keeping up with all the latest hairstyles, and bodies too were becoming increasingly high maintenance. Icons such as Twiggy and Mia Farrow, and the punishing demands of miniskirts and elfin hair cuts, helped fuel the development of the diet industry.

Weight-Watching

Slimming pills were widely available. Amphetamine-based drugs such as Dexedrine or purple hearts were prescribed to housewives wanting to lose weight and filtered through to the youth market, where speed became a favourite recreational drug (particularly associated with Mods). Manufacturers experimented with low calorie foods: Coca-Cola launched TaB, their first sugar-free drink in 1963. The drink was eventually marketed in a pink can designed to appeal to women and the name was inspired by the idea of consumers keeping 'tabs' on their weight (although critics suggested it was an acronym for Totally Artificial Beverage). Doctors devised fashionable diets – the Atkins diet first appeared in *Harper's Bazaar* in 1966, and the following year Dr Irwin Stillman published *The Doctor's Quick Weight Loss Diet*, familiarly known as the water diet, because that was by far the largest constituent. Women's magazines advertised home saunas and vibrating massage machines. Yoga became the latest heath fad.

For thirty-eight-year-old New York housewife Jean Nidetch however nothing seemed to work. She weighed 214lbs and had a history of failed diets when, in September 1961, she invited six overweight friends to join a weekly support group at her house. As the ladies lost weight so the group grew bigger. In 1963 Jean founded Weight Watchers and, by the end of the 1960s, the company had expanded into a multi-million dollar worldwide business. In Britain, once grand country houses were turned into health spas (familiarly known as fat farms) and with the rise of the counter culture, vegetarianism flourished. Cranks, London's first vegetarian restaurant opened in Carnaby Street in 1961, the name a deliberate parody of the nuttiness associated with the health food fad.

Are You Going to San Francisco?

Alternative lifestyle choices also affected fashion and beauty. 1966-7 saw the emergence of the hippies. Beginning in San Francisco the movement expanded across America and Europe; spreading messages of free love and peaceful revolution; popularising mind-expanding drugs ('Turn on, tune in, drop out,' advised LSD guru Timothy Leary); psychedelic music; and rainbow-coloured, flower power fashions.

'The kooky kids of 66 have been replaced by the flower girls of 67. Swinging London is awash with hippie fashion,' reported the *Daily Mirror* during what became known as the Summer of Love.

As kids let it let it all hang out at festivals and love-ins, they put flowers in their hair and drew them on their skin. Body painting became an alternative art movement and permeated into high fashion. The statuesque model Verushka appeared in *Vogue* wearing nothing but

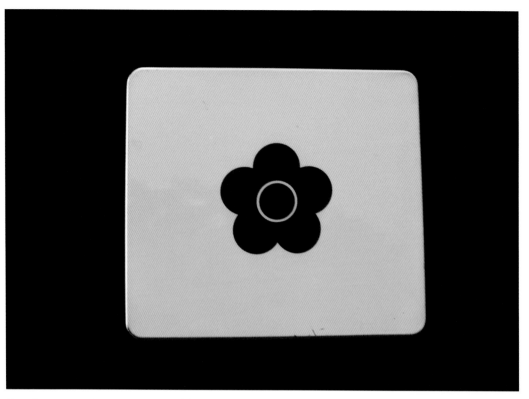

Mary Quant cosmetic crayons – open and closed, c.1970.

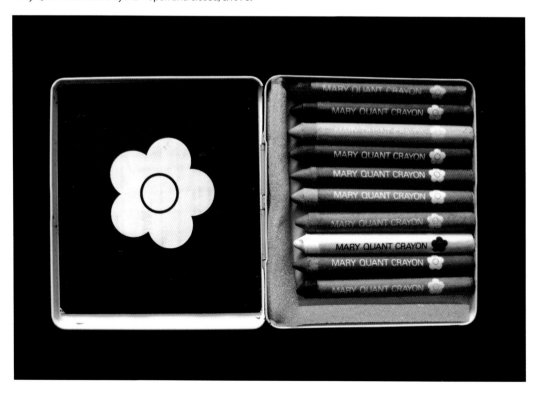

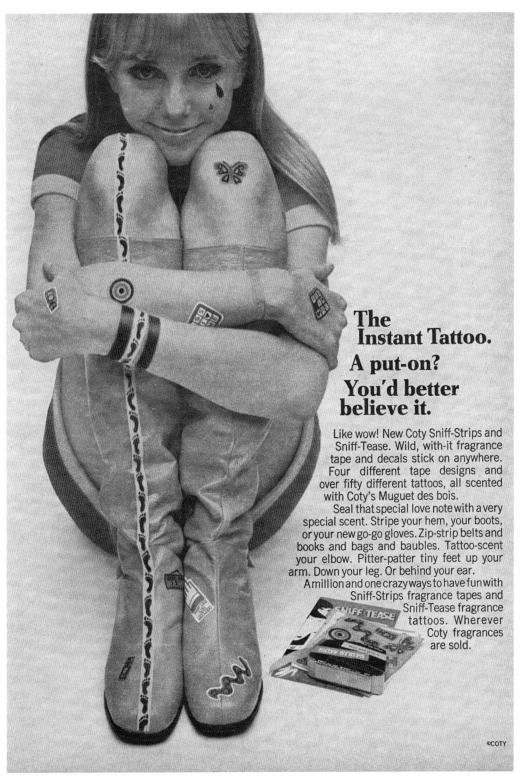

The
Instant Tattoo.
A put-on?
You'd better
believe it.

Like wow! New Coty Sniff-Strips and Sniff-Tease. Wild, with-it fragrance tape and decals stick on anywhere. Four different tape designs and over fifty different tattoos, all scented with Coty's Muguet des bois.

Seal that special love note with a very special scent. Stripe your hem, your boots, or your new go-go gloves. Zip-strip belts and books and bags and baubles. Tattoo-scent your elbow. Pitter-patter tiny feet up your arm. Down your leg. Or behind your ear.

A million and one crazy ways to have fun with Sniff-Strips fragrance tapes and Sniff-Tease fragrance tattoos. Wherever Coty fragrances are sold.

©COTY

1967 Advertisement for Coty Instant Tattoo Sniff-Strips and Sniff-Tease.

patterns drawn over her skin. Inspired by seeing her models colouring their eyes with Caran d'Ache pencils, Mary Quant produced a bright yellow box of cosmetic wax crayons. 'A daisy on ears, stars on your feet … draw crazy patterns and put them wherever you want,' enticed the instructions.

Make-up traditional style was indeed out. Travellers returned from the hippy trail with henna, kohl and patchouli, and experimented with exotic cosmetics along with ethnic textiles, Eastern religions and foreign drugs. Carnaby Street, once the centre of sharp mod styles, became a cultural hotchpotch of smells and bells: the incense-scented boutiques filled with Indian cheesecloth, Peruvian ponchos and Arabian oils. Miniskirts were replaced by long trailing maxi dresses, and short geometric hair cuts by long trailing locks.

Revolutionary Hair

As the swinging sixties evolved into the rioting sixties, what you did to your hair, expressed more than just fashion. 'Who taught you to hate the texture of your hair?' demanded Malcolm X who described the painful and commonplace process of conking (chemically straightening) black hair as the first 'step towards self-degradation'. The Afro was both a style statement and a political one – a symbol of Black Pride and the Black Power movement.

The defining musical of the hippie generation was simply entitled *Hair* (1967). Long hair (particularly when worn by men) was associated with the counterculture. As US youth protested

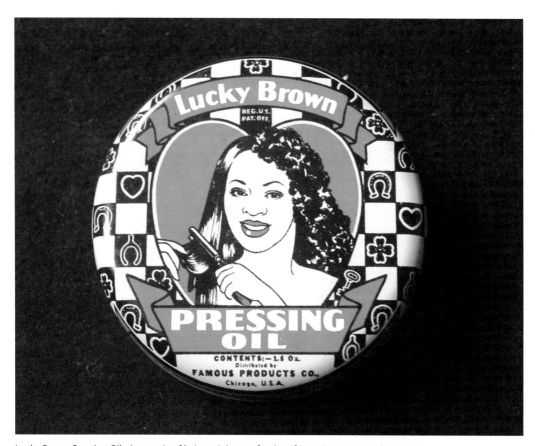

Lucky Brown Pressing Oil, vintage tin of hair straightener for the African-American market, c.1940s.

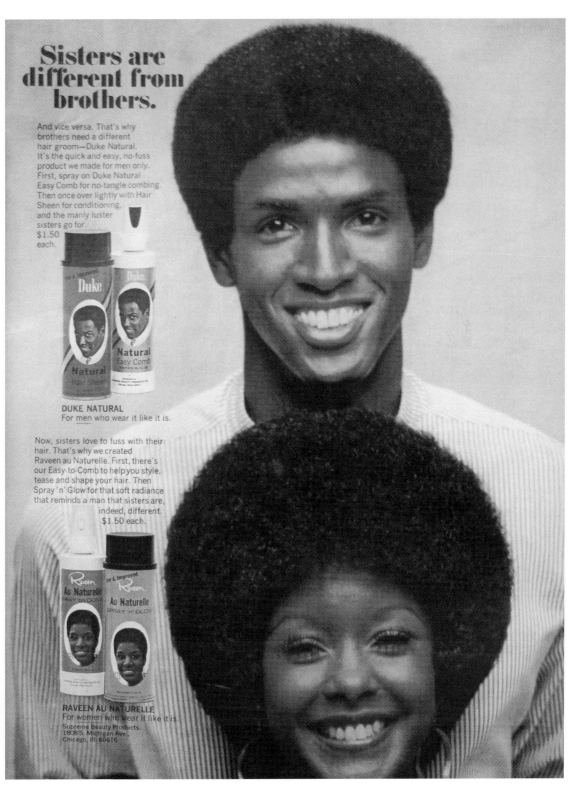

'Sisters are different from brothers' – 1969 advertisement for Duke and Raven hairspray.

against the draft and the Vietnam War it provided an obvious counterpoint to the army crew cut and across the world reflected an anti-establishment position and an instantly recognisable uniform for the children of the revolution. 'Long hair gets people uptight – more uptight than ideology, cause long hair is communication,' observed Jerry Rubin, founder of the Yippies. 'We are a new minority group, a nationwide community of longhairs…Wherever we go, our hair tells people where we stand on Vietnam, Wallace, campus disruption, dope. We're living TV commercials for the revolution. We're walking picket signs.'

Long hair was also a signifier of the sexual revolution. Throughout the sixties men's dress had become increasingly decorative. 'One week he's in polka dots, the next week he's in stripes,' sang The Kinks, chronicling the peacock styles of London's dedicated followers of fashion, who outraged the establishment with their frilly shirts and high-heeled boots. As the sixties drew to a close what with their kaftans, love beads and cascading curls, boys were becoming increasingly indistinguishable from girls: paving the way for the full-blown androgyny of seventies glam, when for the first time since the Eighteenth Century, it was men who wore the prettiest clothes and the most outrageous make-up.

On the Sixties Dressing Table

Although manufacturers tried to keep up with the times, decorating powder compacts with psychedelic flowers and trendy images from The Beatles to the Post Office Tower, as the sixties got into full swing, these little golden boxes appeared increasingly old-fashioned and fuddy-duddy. 'Never have curly gilt or pink plastic. To me they are the antithesis of femininity,' advised Mary Quant in 1968. 'I think you want something that is hard to lose; noticeable in shape, simple but bold in colour.'

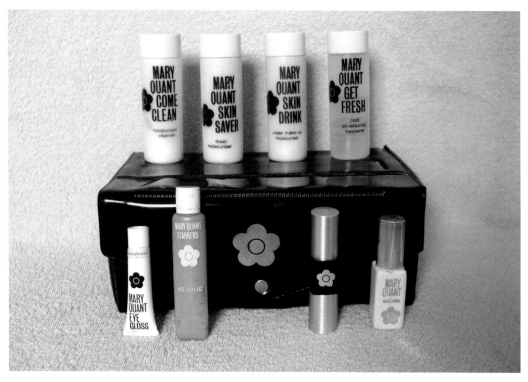

Mary Quant 'The Overnighter' black vinyl beauty box 'Just right for last minute dates straight from work' containing Quant creams and cosmetics.

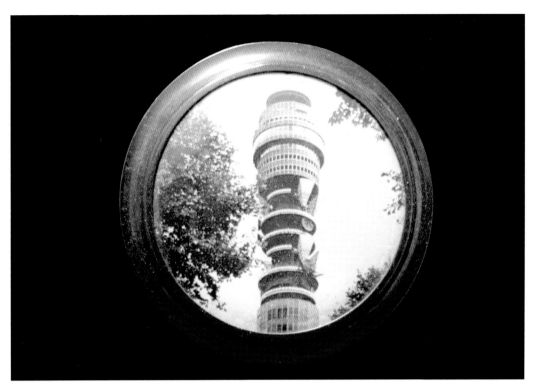

Post Office Tower compact made by Mascot, 1960s.

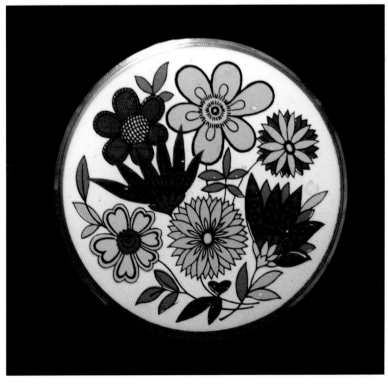

Compact decorated with flowers – unmarked 1960s.

Quant's cosmetics and beauty range (collected by sixties enthusiasts today) came in sleek, mod style packaging accessorised with her trademark daisy motif. Names were direct with a witty twist: Come Clean cleanser, Get Fresh toner, Jeepers Peepers eye gloss. Instructions were presented in strip cartoon form. Make-up bags were made from shiny black and white PVC; face crayons came in a yellow tin, practical, colourful and modern.

'We live in a throwaway economy, a culture in which the most fundamental classification of our ideas and worldly possessions is in terms of their relative expendability,' observed the critic Reyner Banham in an article which was first published in 1960, and popularised the phrase 'throw-away culture' to describe the new mood of galloping consumerism.

In a decade that came up with the paper dress and the blow-up chair, instant gratification was more important than lasting pleasure. Cosmetic companies increasingly gave up on metal containers in favour of plastic: light to carry, colourful to look at, cheap enough to throw away – and of course to buy again.

Packaging designers borrowed from contemporary art movements: plastic containers were decorated with pop-art patterns and psychedelic swirls. Swinging London was a favourite theme. Yardley named lipsticks 'Chelsea Pink' and 'Pinkadilly' and pop art style advertisements told women how to get the 'London Look'. For a new range of make-up launched in 1967 their traditional lavender seller logo was abandoned in favour of Twiggy, who lent her name to false eyelashes and mod-style black and white eye shadows. Yardley's products are sought after by collectors today and in the sixties the brand achieved a cool image (particularly in the USA) that it subsequently struggled to maintain.

In 1968 Boots launched their 17 make-up targeted at the youth market, and teenage fashions had a major influence on beauty products. Miniskirts stimulated a brief craze for leg make-up, including foundation to cover up blemishes, dark powder to slim the legs and liquid rouge for the knees. Coty sniff-strips were pop art style scented tattoos that you could stick over your skin and clothes.

Not since the Edwardian period had false hair been so popular. Wig boxes and styrofoam wig heads were fashionable accessories. Wigs were available everywhere from Woolworths to Harrods and by the late 1960s the UK wig industry was worth £13 million a year.

False eyelashes came in every material from mink to human hair and at the height of flower power girls stuck sequins on their eyelids and coloured their faces with wax crayons and poster paints. 'God knows what it would do to your skin because it's got lead in it,' winced Twiggy.

Yet at the same time cosmetic companies and their customers were becoming increasingly sophisticated. In 1966 Revlon came up with

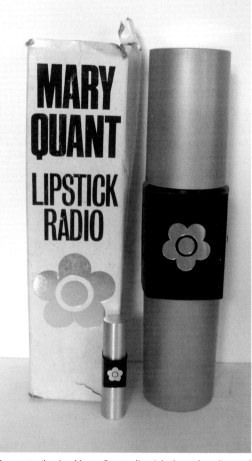

Pop art classic: Mary Quant lipstick-shaped radio and lipstick, 1960s.

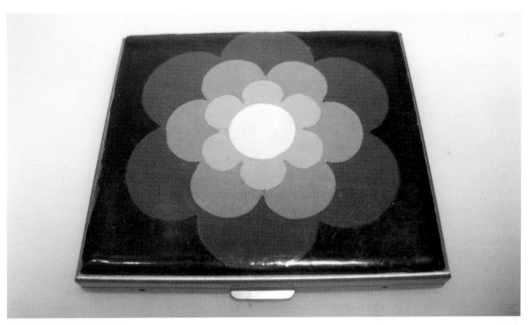

1960s compact decorated with a Mary Quant style flower in brown, black and white enamel. *Gray's Antiques*

Natural wonder, 'The first total collection of medicated make-up and treatments designed especially for young, unpredictable skin.' Two years later saw the establishment of Clinique (an offshoot of the Estée Lauder Company), its fragrance free, allergy-tested skincare products targeted at individuals rather than offering one cream to suit all needs.

'Beauty is growing up,' observed *Queen* Magazine in 1968. 'Girls who used to be enticed at the beauty counter by names like 'Glamour Glow' and 'Magic Moonbeams' are now more likely to ask for the new cream with leichol or triglycerides.' From the sixties onwards cosmetics firms increasingly seduced their customers with science, the simplest ingredients being given the most complex names. As the Twentieth Century progressed tighter regulations might have obliged manufacturers to identify the contents of their products, but with many of the words used seemingly extracted from the Scrabble dictionary, purchasers were often left little wiser than before about what they were putting on their faces.

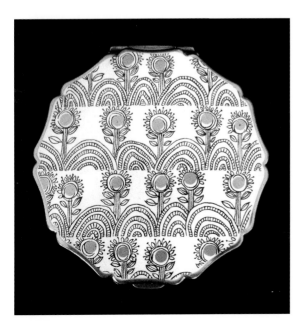

1960s black, white and gold enamel compact by Stratton.

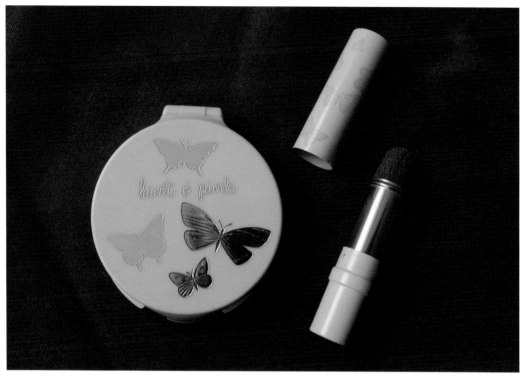

'Hint o' Pink' compact and powder brush; Fuller Brush Company USA, 1962.

Boxed set of Pond's Angel Face eye make-up available from *Woman* Magazine, early 1960s.

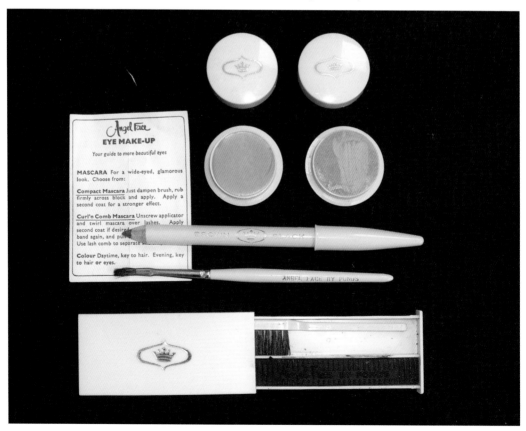

CHAPTER TEN

Glam Men and Hairy Women

Beauty in the 1970s

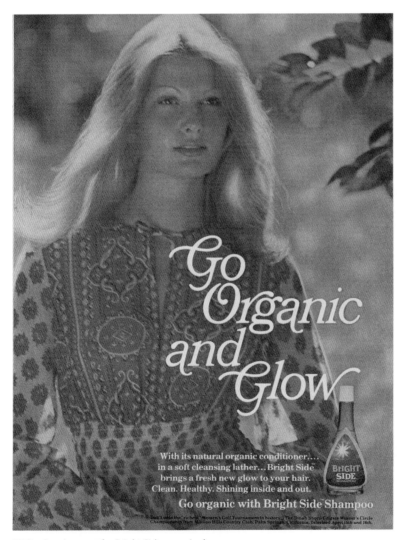

1972 advertisement for Bright Side organic shampoo.

F THE SIXTIES looked forward to a brave new world epitomised by shiny space age fashions and the Apollo moon landing, then the seventies turned back to a romantic, decorative past.

There was a distinct mood of nostalgia. The TV drama series *Upstairs Downstairs* (1971–75), chronicling the lives and loves of an Edwardian family and their servants, was watched by over a billion people in seventy countries across the world. *The Country Diary of an Edwardian Lady* – illustrated by an amateur naturalist in 1906 – became the publishing sensation of 1977, selling 3 million copies and launching an avalanche of merchandise. Edwardian Lady tins and floral tea towels were perfect accessories for the stripped pine, farmhouse-style kitchens that became a seventies favourite even in the most urban homes.

Fashion and beauty reflected the spirit of revivalism. Crabtree and Evelyn might have sounded like an ancient British apothecary, in fact it was a new American company, founded in Massachusetts in 1973, the name and retro packaging of soaps and lotions a deliberate attempt to conjure up visions of 'ye olde England', a country cottage garden, and a rosy-cheeked peaches and cream complexion. Boots rose oil came in a Victorian style brown glass bottle, housed in a miniature wicker picnic basket.

Retro Girls

The Victorian/Edwardian look was in. The girls of swinging London swapped miniskirts and Vidal Sassoon bobs for natural flowing curls and long Laura Ashley dresses. 'I looked like Holly Hobbie!' remembers one former seventies teenager. 'I also had Laura Ashley curtains in my bedroom, and if I stood against them in one of my milkmaid frocks, I practically disappeared.'

Rather than being inspired by street style and man-made fibres, Laura Ashley explored the costume collections at the Victoria and Albert Museum, and revived vintage chintzes and sprigged cottons. It was a fresh-faced look and, while the company was eventually to introduce fragrances, make-up was not part of their mighty empire, which by 1975 was turning over £5 million per annum. The Ashley image was pretty but it wasn't exactly sexy; for a more glamorous vision of the past (and more cosmetics than a girl could dream of) you had to go to Biba.

Barbara Hulanicki started Biba (named after her sister) as a small mail order business, selling cheap and cheerful teenage fashions. In 1964 she opened a tiny boutique in Kensington and Biba became the Mecca for swinging London. Everyone, from pop stars to secretaries, squeezed into London's first communal changing rooms to try on art deco inspired clothes, fluffy feather boas, and skin-tight suede boots in Biba's distinctive sludgy palette; brown, plum, mulberry and grape – the colours of bruised, overripe fruit.

Business boomed and Biba expanded into ever-larger premises, culminating in their final move to the former Derry and Toms building on Kensington High Street in 1973. Hulanicki transformed the neglected 1930s department store into an art deco pleasure palace lined with marble, draped with leopard skin and illuminated with dark, atmospheric lighting that was a gift to shoplifters, who visited the store in their thousands. The famous Rainbow Room restaurant looked like cross between a Hollywood film set and thirties ocean liner; the roof garden was home to penguins and pink flamingos. 'Walk into the new Biba,' enthused the *Evening News*, 'and you'll feel as if you've stepped inside a dream machine.'

With six enormous floors to fill, Hulanicki expanded her range to sell everything from baked beans to bed sheets but perhaps her most successful line of all was cosmetics.

Biba make-up was launched in 1970 in typical retro style, with a 1930s tea dance, a life-size cake in the shape of a Biba cosmetics girl and a bevy of slender beauties wafting round in flowing crepe – smoky-eyed, spiky-lashed and chocolate-lipped. It was a radical new look. 'Wherever the girls went there was silence,' remembered Hulanicki. 'Elly was completely blue: blue make-up, blue clothes, blue cap and blue curls. Eva was all green, Del all violet. Some girls were all in black, looking like Dracula.' Moving away from traditional pinks, corals and reds, Hulanicki's make-up was in the same distinctive dusky colours as her clothes; black, mahogany, purple, pewter … presaging the Goth look and creating a high camp thirties glamour, emphasised by the signature black and gold packaging.

Art deco style make-up became all the rage; pioneered by Hulanicki, and promoted in fashionable films of the day from *The Boyfriend* (featuring a new 1920s style Twiggy) to *Cabaret*. 'Imagine you've been chosen to play Daisy in *The Great Gatsby*,' advised *Vogue* helpfully in 1973, recommending plums and violets for the eyes and 'a rosebud 20s mouth'. It was a self-consciously theatrical style that required some practice. Biba's deco mirrored make-up counters were filled with dozens of testers – another innovation: 'We were the first to encourage customers to experiment before they bought,' claimed Hulanicki in her autobiography. 'Some even came in very early in the morning with faces scrubbed clean, and made themselves up and continued on to work.'

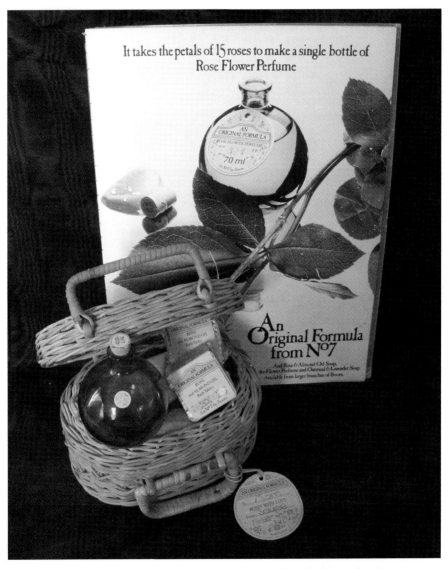

Boots No. 7 original formula rose oil and bathcube set with original 1977 advertisement.

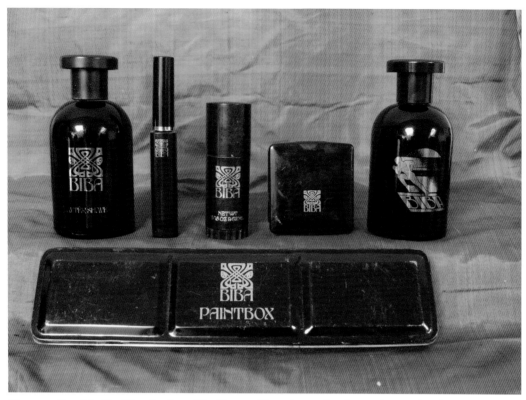

Biba cosmetics : 2 bottles Biba aftershave; Biba Mascara; Biba twist up silver face make-up; Biba plastic eye make-up compact; Biba Paintbox – tinplate eye shadow container, 1970s.

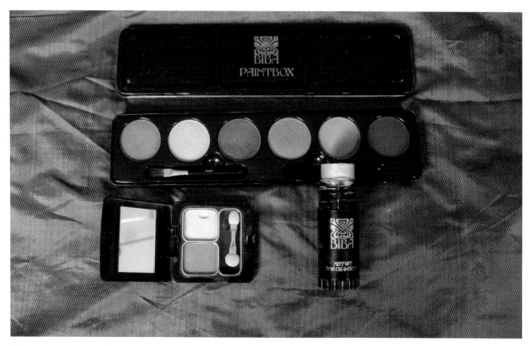

Biba cosmetics open, showing the classic Biba make-up Palette.

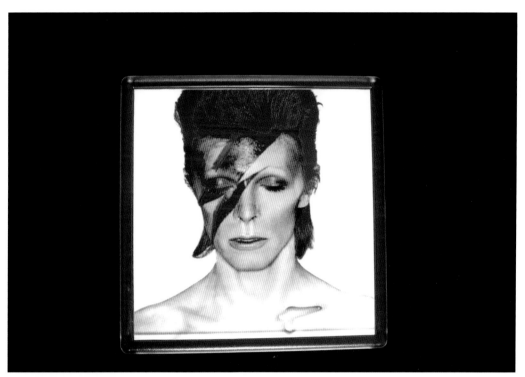

Modern make-up mirror showing David Bowie in Aladdin Sane make-up c.1973.

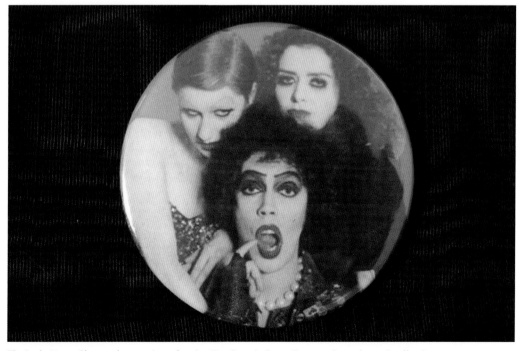

The Rocky Horror Show make-up mirror showing Tim Curry in Sweet Transvestite make-up (modern).

Glam Men

It wasn't just girls playing with make-up in the early seventies. This was the age of Glam. Lou Reed and Freddy Mercury both sported Biba's black nail varnish. The most extravagantly made-up figures of the period were undoubtedly the boys: Mark Bolan in his glitter eye make-up and feather boa; David Bowie as Ziggy Stardust and Aladdin Sane; and Tim Curry as Frank'N'Furter, star of *The Rocky Horror Show*, who stunned London theatre in audiences 1973, when he sashayed on to the stage in fishnet stockings, high heels, satin basque and full on 'sweet transvestite' slap.

The androgyny of early glam offered a decorative reflection of new attitudes to sexuality. In Britain the Sexual Offences Bill passed in 1967 had legalised gay sex in private between consenting adults over the age of twenty-one, and in America the Stonewall riots of 1969 led to the founding of the Gay Liberation Movement.

As homosexuals came out of the closet so did clothes and make-up formerly restricted to women. David Bowie appeared in a dress on the UK album cover of *The Man Who Sold The World*

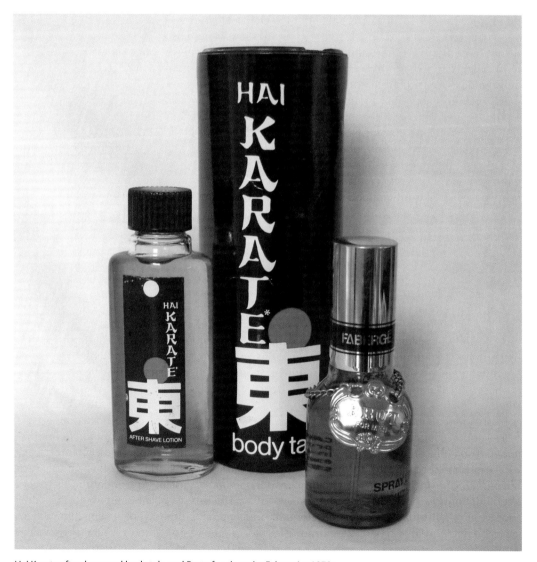

Hai Karate aftershave and body talc, and Brut aftershave by Fabergé, c.1970s.

(1970) and declared his bisexuality to the press (a statement he later retracted). The Ziggy look ('a cross between Nijinsky and Woolworths,' explained Bowie) seduced scores of fans gay and straight alike who adopted the bright red rooster hair cut and the zigzag Aladdin Sane face paint. Seeing pretty young men in make-up on *Top of the Pops* was not only a defining rock and roll moment, but for some offered a first view of an alternative lifestyle. Holly Johnson, Boy George, Marc Almond are just some of the gay pop stars of the eighties, who cite Bowie and glam rock as a formative influence on their work and lives. 'Glam rock was cheap, trashy and kitsch – and for a brief moment, it offered a lifeline to a boy on the brink of adolescence and unsure of his own sexuality,' novelist Jake Arnott told *The Observer* (April 23, 2006).

Though it never lost its campness, as it stomped on silver platforms into the seventies, glam was not just about androgyny. All the glitter make-up in the world couldn't make seventies British bands like Slade or Mud appear remotely feminine: 'Bricklayers in drag,' sneered one commentator. In the USA, Alice Cooper might have flaunted a girl's name and more cosmetics than Superdrug, but their act was famous for its theatrically masculine violence. Even if they never actually beheaded chickens on stage, they looked as though they might. US supergroup Kiss modelled their outrageous make-up on cartoon superheroes, eventually spawning vast amounts of profitable merchandise including a Kiss make-up kit, and their own Marvel comic book; the original illustrations allegedly drawn with drops of the band members' blood.

Whether gay or straight, stylish, silly, or ostentatiously sick, glam legitimised make-up for men and confirmed it as part of the rock and roll armoury. Growing interest in male toiletries filtered down to the civilian population. 'According to recent statistics approximately £8 million a year is spent on men's cosmetics,' reported *Harpers & Queen* in February 1973. The fashion for big hair (Kevin Keegan curls, Hendrix Afros, Bowie mullets) and for facial hair (sideburns and handlebar moustaches) fuelled demand for grooming products. Sales of aftershave boomed; popular brands included Hai Karate, which originally came packaged with a self-defence leaflet for dealing with women driven mad by your fragrance, and most famously Brut by Fabergé – the archetypal smell of seventies man. The butch name and advertisements featuring boxer Henry Cooper emphasised the fact that wearing perfume wouldn't turn you into a 'pouf' and the chained metal label mirrored the male fashion for wearing medallions.

Hairy Women

While men embraced beauty products in the seventies one sector of the female population was advised to reject them almost entirely.

For the burgeoning Women's Movement cosmetics represented female subjugation by an oppressive patriarchal society. The women's liberationists who picketed the Miss America contest in 1968 tossed bras and make-up into a 'Freedom trash can' (fuelling popular myths about bra burning). Gloria Steinem told women that anybody who spent more than fifteen minutes getting ready in the morning was 'getting screwed'. Feminist writers denounced stereotypes of female beauty and traditional feminine grooming practices. 'I'm sick of pretending eternal youth. I'm sick of belying my own intelligence, my own will, my own sex. I'm sick of peering at the world through false eyelashes … I'm sick of the powder room,' raged Germaine Greer in the *Female Eunuch* (1970). 'Every day, in every way the billion dollar beauty business tells women they are monsters in disguise,' warned Una Stannard in the *Mask of Beauty* (1971). 'Every ad for bras tells women that her breasts need lifting … every ad for cosmetics that her skin is too dry, too oily, too pale, or too ruddy, that her lips are not bright enough or her lashes not long enough; every ad for deodorants and perfumes that her natural odours all need disguising.'

Shaving armpits and legs was equated with the suppression of female sexuality, and depilation was generally discouraged. 'KEEP YOUR HAIR ON – ALL OF IT …' advised *Nova* magazine in October 1971, over a double page picture of a nude woman with defiantly tufty pubic hair.

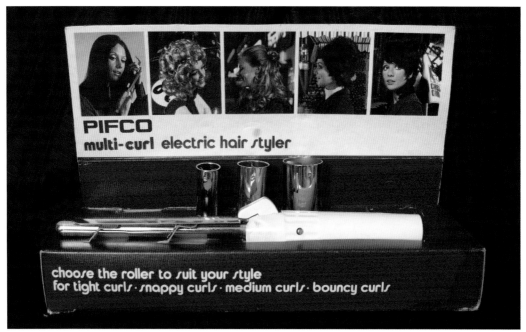

Pifco multi-curl electric hair styler, c.1972.

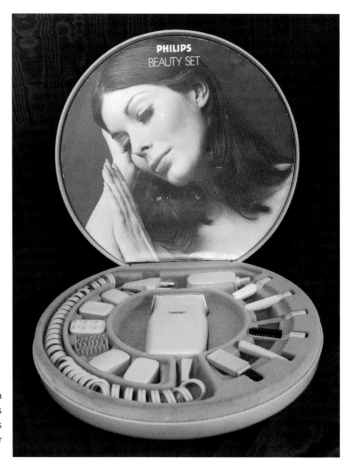

Philips Beauty Set 1970s. Most women however stuck to the shaving ritual. This Philips beauty set in classic seventies orange plastic, includes attachments for shaving, massage and manicure.

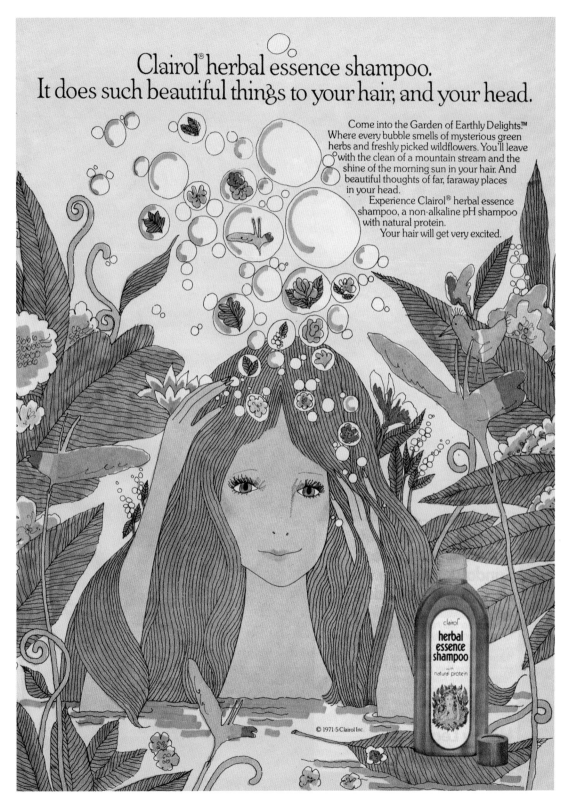

1970s advertisement for Clairol Herbal Essence Shampoo.

Hippie Chicks

The hippie movement also rejected mass-produced cosmetics and images of manicured beauty. 'We didn't wear make-up – at least we weren't really supposed to,' remembers one English girl who followed The Grateful Dead to San Francisco, where she lived in a hippie commune in the early seventies. 'It was all very hands on and artsy-crafty. There was a lot of interest in mixing your own creams from natural products and essential oils. We made our own soap and scented candles and there was a local store called the Body Shop where you could take in bottles to be filled with shampoos and oils. People think recycling and being green is very Twenty-first Century, but it's exactly what we were doing thirty years ago.'

At the same period Anita Roddick hit the hippie trail and travelled the world. 'I saw raw ingredients being used as they had been for centuries, to polish the skin, to cleanse the hair and to protect both,' she remembered. Inspired by traditional cosmetics from across the globe and by the Californian prototype, Roddick opened her own Body Shop in Brighton in 1976. Though she started with only twenty natural-based products, they came in five different sized plastic bottles, both to make the shop look fuller and to allow customers to buy as much or as little as they wanted. Walls were painted green (later the signature Body Shop colour) to cover up damp patches. Lack of money led to no advertising, minimal packaging and refillable containers with handwritten labels. Through a combination of financial necessity and personal passion the Body Shop's green philosophy was born.

The Body Shop's avowed mission statement was to protect the planet and conserve natural resources, but ironically one of the reasons it became so successful was the increasing mass consumption of cosmetics in the 1970s. As more women entered the workplace, so demand for beauty products boomed. Revlon's sales figures went from around $314 million in 1971 to £606 million in 1974, reflecting both the burgeoning market and the worldwide success of Charlie launched in 1973 – the smell of seventies women.

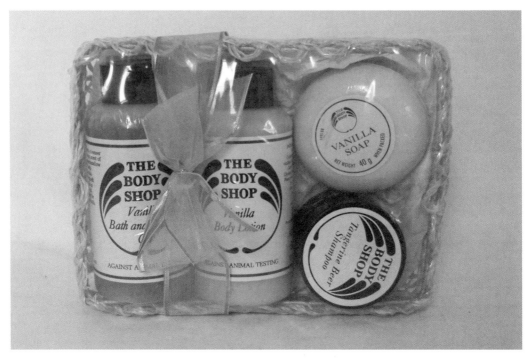

Vintage Body Shop gift set.

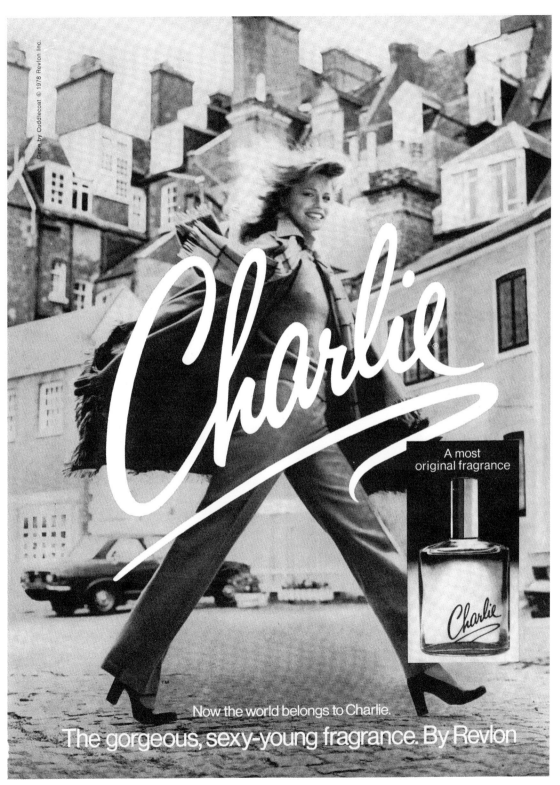

Charlie Fragrance Advertisment, 1970s.

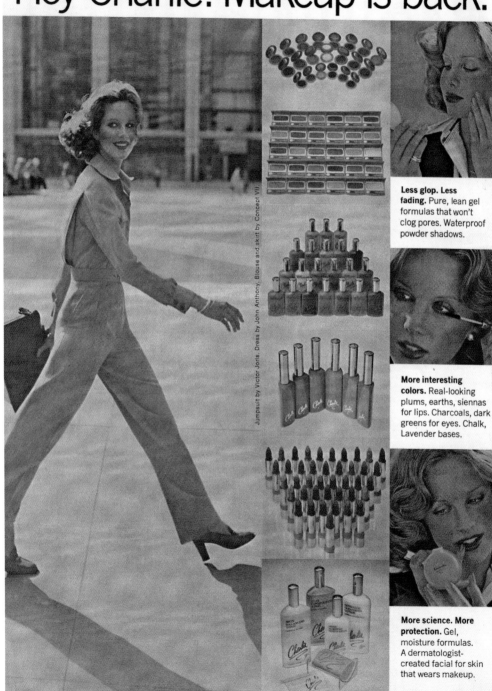

Hey Charlie! Makeup is back.

Jumpsuit by Victor Joris. Dress by John Anthony. Blouse and skirt by Concept VII

Less glop. Less fading. Pure, lean gel formulas that won't clog pores. Waterproof powder shadows.

More interesting colors. Real-looking plums, earths, siennas for lips. Charcoals, dark greens for eyes. Chalk, Lavender bases.

More science. More protection. Gel, moisture formulas. A dermatologist-created facial for skin that wears makeup.

Charlie make-up advertisement, 1970s.

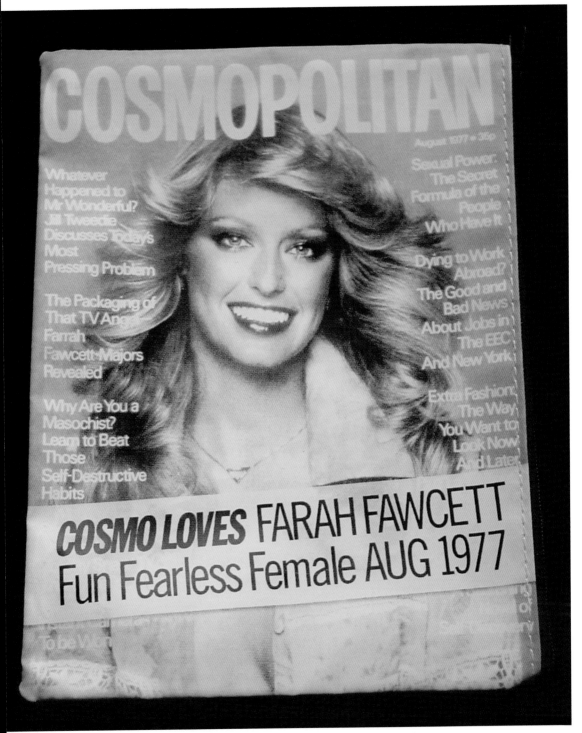

Vintage Farrah Fawcett make-up bag showing 1977 *Cosmo* Cover.

Charlie Girls

Described as 'the first feminist fragrance', Revlon's new perfume was code-named Cosmo during its development, indicating its target audience: working women under the age of thirty; the young, liberated readers of the hugely successful *Cosmopolitan* magazine.

Founded in the USA in 1886, *Cosmopolitan* magazine was revolutionised in the second half of the 1960s by editor Helen Gurley Brown (author of the best selling book *Sex and the Single Girl*), who captured the mood and aspirations of a new generation. Articles on home decoration and babies were out; features on sex, work and beauty were in.

'You are that Cosmopolitan girl, aren't you?' demanded the editorial of the first issue of British *Cosmopolitan* magazine, launched in 1972. 'You're very interested in men, naturally, but think too much of yourself to live your life entirely through him. That means you're going to make the most of yourself – your body, your face, your clothes, your hair, your job and your mind.'

Charlie captured this new mood of independence and was marketed as a scent that women could buy for themselves. The name (inspired by Charles Revson) was androgynous, but sexy and sassy. Advertisements featured models in trousers (almost unheard of in perfume publicity) striding confidently forward in their Ralph Lauren clothes – relaxed and sure of themselves whether at work or at play.

Revlon wasn't just selling fragrance and cosmetics, but a lifestyle, and the image representing that lifestyle became increasingly important. Revlon was the first company to offer a model an exclusive contract to represent their products when in 1973 Lauren Hutton became the face of Ultima II Make-up, with a contract beginning at $175,000 for thirty-five days' work. Two years later Margaux Hemingway received a record $1 million to become the face of Fabergé's Babe beauty range, and thanks to the giant cosmetic companies, the 1970s saw the creation of the super rich, supermodel.

The healthy American look – fresh face, sparkling eyes, sun-kissed skin, lots of shiny hair and lots of dazzling white teeth – was everywhere in magazines and on television and was epitomised by another Charlie girl; Farah Fawcett-Majors, star of the popular US TV series *Charlie's Angels* (1976). Farah was the archetypal American seventies blonde and a marketing sensation. For little girls there were Farah dolls. For women there was Fabergé's Farah Fawcett Shampoo (and many misspent hours at the hairdressers imitating her feather-cut, tousled mane). For men there was a poster which, showing Farah in a red swimsuit, demonstrated why *Charlie's Angels* popularised the expression 'Jiggle TV', and shifting a reported 12 million copies became the best-selling poster of all time.

Punk

But not everybody wanted to buy into the Californian dream. 'If you give me the chance, I'll destroy America for you,' snarled Johnny Rotten, lead singer of the Sex Pistols. Punk, emerging in mid-seventies Britain from a period of recession, disenchantment and bad dentistry, offered a radically alternative look.

Clothes, hair and make-up were as important to the punk movement as music, and were just as anarchic. Vivienne Westwood and Malcolm McLaren's shop in London's King's Road; opened in 1971 as Let it Rock; renamed Too Fast to Live, too Young to Die in 1972; and then Sex in 1974; was the centre of punk fashion. The provocatively-named and scary looking store was the source of bondage trousers, obscene T-shirts and the birthplace of the Sex Pistols, managed by McLaren, and so-called in part to advertise the shop (until its name was changed again in 1977 to Seditionaries) as well as to stick two fingers up to the world at large. Both visually and musically punks set out to shock the establishment and challenge traditional notions of beauty. 'We made ugliness beautiful,' recalled McLaren. 'It was wonderful to sell something that was horrible.'

Hair was dyed rampantly artificial colours – jet black, peroxide blond, neon pink, mouldy green … anything as long as it didn't look natural. Styles ranged from razor short crops to, as the movement progressed, huge gelled spikes and day-glo Mohicans. Make-up was inspired by the vampire look: pale skin (aided and abetted by drink, drugs, and an urban, indoor lifestyle), black painted lips and eyes, and occasionally patterns and symbols scrawled across the face. 'The make-up is armour. It's tribal, primal. It's still war paint,' explained singer Siouxsie Sioux in a recent interview.

Punk style was perhaps most famously modelled by Jordan – shop assistant at Sex and star of Derek Jarman's 1978 film *Jubilee* – who when she commuted by train from Sussex in black rubber bondage gear, peroxide beehive and abstract face paint, created such a stir that British Rail put her in a first-class carriage for her own safety.

Jamie Reid's 1977 picture of the Queen with a safety pin through her lip – part of the art work designed for the Sex Pistols *God Save the Queen* single – became one of the most iconic images of the period. As with clothes, punks borrowed skin decoration from the fetish and biker scenes, pioneering the tattooing and piercing that were to become commonplace twenty years later.

Though punk was deliberately anti-fashion and courted controversy, it soon became mainstream. The bondage-trousered, spiky-haired kids in the King's Road were one of the sights of London. Tourist shops sold postcards of leering punks alongside pictures of Beefeaters, both epitomising a British taste for eccentricity and dressing up. Fashion designers from Zandra Rhodes to Versace experimented with torn clothing and gilded safety pins, and Vivienne Westwood went on to become the leading British couturier of the late Twentieth Century. Thanks to punk, by the end of the decade, and to the dismay of many parents, single earrings, eyeliner and dyed hair were commonly worn by young men.

Punk was an aggressive visual style, but paradoxically it was also democratic. You didn't have to be rich to dress like a punk. Although you could buy your Vivienne Westwood originals at considerable expense from Sex; you could also do it yourself with a bin liner, a ripped T-shirt, a magic marker and a kohl pencil. The movement certainly had its great beauties (Siouxsie Sioux and Debbie Harry were the ultimate punk pin-ups) but because punk was deliberately ugly it embraced unattractiveness. Physical imperfections could even accessorise your look. Poly Styrene, lead singer of X-Ray Spex, made a feature of her braces; Shane McGowan, founder of the Nipple Erectors and then the Pogues, became famous for his lack of teeth. In much the same way as you didn't have to play an instrument to be in a band, so you didn't have to be pretty to be a punk – and frankly if you were sporting a lime green Mohawk hairdo, a safety pin through your nose and a T-shirt emblazoned with swastikas and a giant penis: who was going to notice what you looked like underneath?

Punk took make-up back to its warpaint roots, separating it from notions of concealment and self-improvement – and using it as a badge of tribal belonging and a declaration of war against the 'fascist regime': a world of conservatism and extravagant consumerism that was to return with a vengeance in the 1980s.

On The Seventies Dressing Table

'To most girls under 25, powder is the stuff their mothers wear,' observed *Harpers & Queen* in 1970. Faced with changing fashions, many compact manufacturers either switched production lines, or simply went out of business. The following year when the magazine ran a feature on the trendy teenage dressing table there wasn't a gilded powder compact in sight or indeed a dressing table. The teenager's cosmetics were displayed on a plastic Habitat wall-unit and included Kiku perfume by Fabergé, Mary Quant's paint box and crayon set and a selection of Biba make-up.

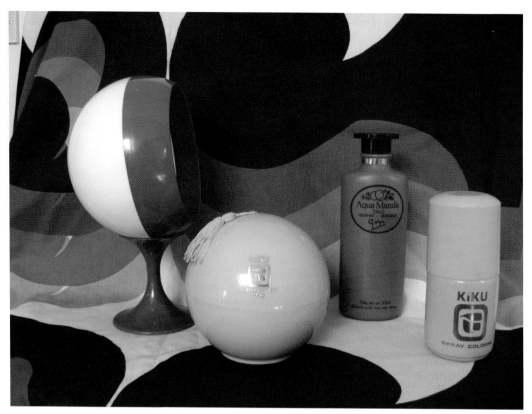

Space age style plastic mirror, orange front unscrews to reveal a makeup box; Kiku dusting powder; Aqua Manda talc, by Goya; Kiku spray cologne, 1970s.

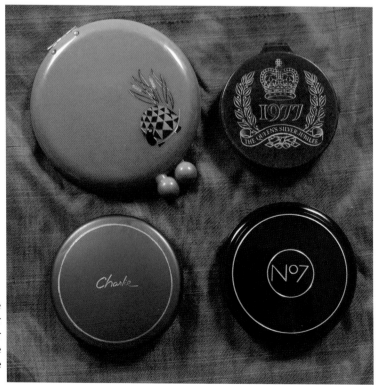

1970s plastic compacts: orange Love-Pat compact; 1977 Silver Jubilee compact for Max Factor Creme Puff; Boots No.7 Creme Touch compact; Charlie face powder compact by Revlon.

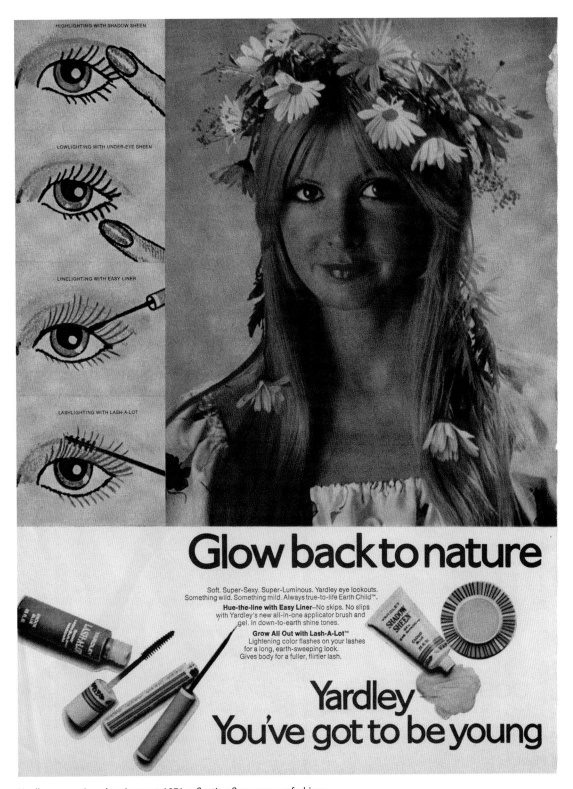

Yardley cosmetics advertisement, 1971, reflecting flower power fashions.

Space age designs and strong pop art colours were popular for period beauty accessories – Kiku's dusting powder came in a bright yellow globe, plastic was the common medium for compacts. Orange, brown, green and yellow were typical packaging colours for bath and beauty products; toning in perfectly with that other seventies favourite – the avocado bathroom suite.

The retro revival was a major influence on the dressing table. Biba cosmetics (much sought after by collectors today) were distinctively packaged in art deco style black and gold and modern beauty products were decorated with vintage graphics.

Biba epitomised the age of glam and the hedonism of the early seventies but with the Oil Crisis of 1973 came unemployment, soaring inflation, and a period of economic chaos. In 1975 Biba went bust, and even make-up reflected the mood of recession. The new look, according to social commentator Peter York was Economy Chic, 'Girls have been wondering round this winter looking like a dosser's bed,' he observed gloomily. 'Economy Chic is essentially reactionary. It is a reaction against the optimism of the sixties and the extravagance of the early seventies ... The mood is one of atonement.'

The natural look was in. Girls experimented with home-made creams and face washes. Indian henna was a popular hair dye; patchouli oil was a hippie favourite – said to mask the smell of cannabis, although many assumed the powerful odour was simply unwashed body. Matching growing interest in whole foods, natural products (oatmeal, milk, etc.) appeared in mass-manufactured cosmetics. Revlon's Natural Beauty Mask (1973) included honey, egg and mint and was advertised by a photograph of a healthy young hippy in headband and ethnic shirt. Shampoo ingredients read like recipe books, filled with fruit, vegetables and herbs.

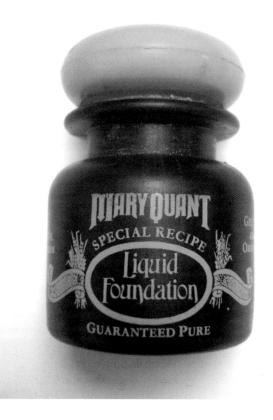

This 1970s plastic bottle of Mary Quant liquid foundation includes honey, almond and wheatgerm oil. Part of Quant's Special Recipe range, it reflects growing interest by cosmetics firms in using natural ingredients.

At The Body Shop Anita Roddick dispensed with superfluous packaging, housing her natural-based beauty products in cheap refillable bottles. Along with growing concern for the environment (presaging the green revolution of the fin de siecle) there was a new interest in alternative remedies. Healer and massage therapist Robert Tisserand started the Aromatic Oil Company in 1974 from the bedroom of his London home. Tisserand's *The Art of Aromatherapy* (1977) was the first English book on the subject and became a standard work of reference.

Not everything natural was good for you. With the fashion for a healthy outdoor look and a bronzed skin, sun tanning became increasingly popular. Period sun care products such as Bergasol provided a dark and quick tan rather than a safe one; frying in Johnson's baby oil, or olive oil was another holiday option. In 1972, West German scientist Friedrich Wolff isolated ultraviolet A (UVA) rays, which tanned rather than burned, and pioneered the indoor tanning industry, selling sun lamp and sun beds first in Europe then, from 1978, in the States. It wasn't until that same year that the US Food and Drug Administration (FDA) confirmed the importance of sunscreens and developed a rating system for SPFs (sun protection factor). For many however it was too late and the 1980s saw a marked increase in cases of skin cancer.

Punks were among the few who didn't want a holiday in the sun, and proudly flaunted their urban pallor, accentuated by black make-up. For those who wanted to experiment with the look, before committing themselves more permanently or painfully, dressing table accessories included Crazy Colour hairspray, transfer tattoos and clip-on safety pins, which could be attached to the nose without piercing.

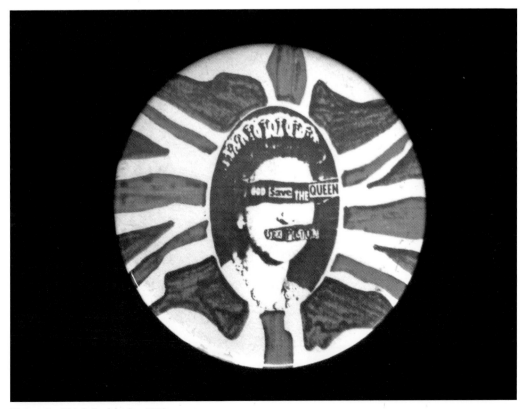

Vintage Sex Pistols Punk badge, 1970s.

CHAPTER ELEVEN

Material Girls and Boys

Beauty in the 1980s

T HE 1980s were a decade of big business, conspicuous consumption and showing off. Madonna proclaimed that we were all living in a material world and the material mood of the moment was epitomised by the vogue for power dressing. Whereas youth culture in the sixties and seventies had sought to escape the fashions and formalities of the adult world, the yuppies of the eighties embraced and exaggerated them. Office suits came with huge padded shoulders, frilled

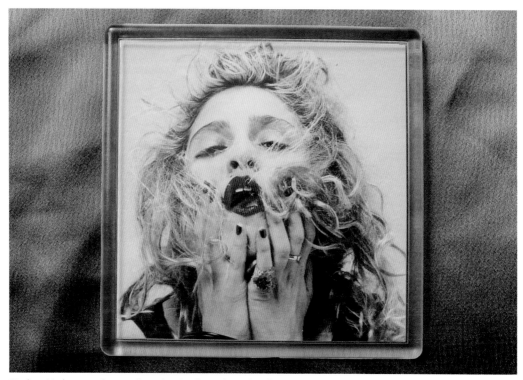

Modern Madonna make-up mirror showing her at her colourful 1980s best.

Split, chipped problem nails?

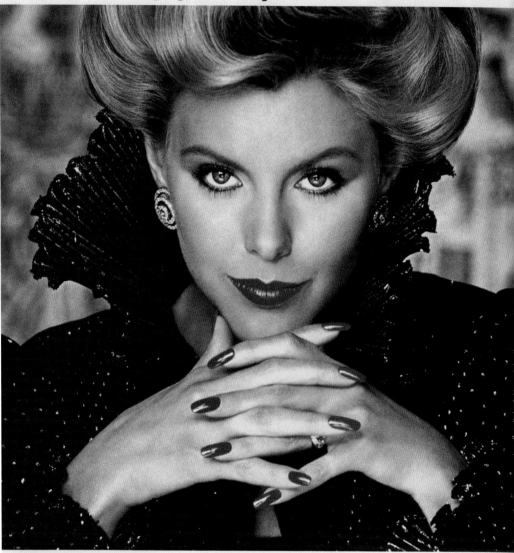

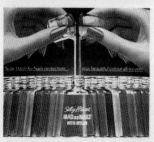

With 'Hard-As-Nails'
patented long-wearing formula,
you get the protection you need
in the colours you want.

Hard-As-Nails with nylon helps strengthen
and helps prevent splitting, cracking,
chipping, breaking or peeling. And with
Hard-As-Nails, protection can be beautiful
in the most exciting colours imaginable.

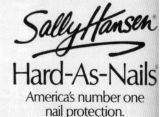

Hard-As-Nails
America's number one
nail protection.

Available in the Republic of Ireland.

Vintage advertisement for Sally Hansen's Hard as Nails showing classic 1980s make-up.

and ruched taffeta ball gowns looked like mobile meringues, and power clothing was matched by power grooming and fragranced with power perfumes.

Big shoulder pads were counterbalanced by big hair – permed, moussed, gelled and flicked, to astonishing volume, and that was just the boys. Shiny materials – which appeared everywhere from suits to Lycra leotards – were complemented by shiny cosmetics; shimmering skin bronzer; bright eye shadow (several shades often worn together); and strong, glossy lipstick. Favourite colours of the decade, both in fashion and cosmetics, included electric blue, fuchsia pink and tomato red, heavily accented with gold – the colour of money, gilt buttons and the blonde highlights, sported by everybody from Madonna to Margaret Thatcher.

Glamour was in, subtlety was out, and whether you were Princess Diana, Boy George or Alexis from Dynasty, high maintenance grooming was essential.

Dress for success

In the decade that gave birth to the yuppie (young urban upwardly-mobile professional) more women entered the boardroom, and what to wear to the office became increasingly important. Britain's first woman prime minister, Margaret Thatcher, pioneered the art of power dressing, mixing the masculine and feminine. 'She has the eyes of Caligula with the mouth of Marilyn Monroe,' observed French President Francois Mitterrand. For women the archetypal eighties suit was composed of padded shouldered jacket and a skirt that showed off the legs. Colours were often bright (Mrs Thatcher favoured Tory blue, Nancy Regan bright red) and accessories were ostentatiously female; large sparkly lapel brooches, a blouse with a pussy cat bow, a statement handbag. Being given a dressing down by the Prime Minister became known in the eighties as 'being handbagged'. The 'Iron Lady' wore her clothes like armour, and hair and make-up were equally invincible. Celebrated cosmetic artist Joan Price advised her on make-up; hairdresser John of Thurloe Place was in constant attendance. As Mrs Thatcher's career progressed, so her hairstyle became bigger and blonder. Detractors dubbed it the 'Bouffant Terrible' and even on an official visit to the Falklands the PM packed her heated rollers.

And who could blame her? In a world of expanding media – more television stations, more magazines and 'lifestyle supplements' featuring beautiful people in their beautiful homes (*Hello!* magazine was launched in 1988) – image was all important and looking good was part of the job. In the USA two former film actors brought a sense of Hollywood glitz to the White House, luxuriously restoring both the interiors and themselves. Nancy Regan was much criticised for spending $210,399 on a new state dinner service decorated in her favourite red and gold and for 'borrowing' designer clothes worth a small fortune (in 1988 *Time* magazine estimated the value of her wardrobe at over $1 million). The first lady's stretched smile and unblinking eyes suggested that her face too had undergone some considerable renovation and though he always denied using dye, the President's hair was surprisingly dark for a man in his seventies.

Greed is Good

If the eighties were characterised by lust for power, money and surface glamour then America was its spiritual home. 'Greed, for lack of a better word, is good. Greed is right,' claimed Gordon Gekko (played by Michael Douglas) corrupt tycoon of the 1987 film *Wall Street* – who with his shiny suit, stripy braces and slicked back hair captured the rapacious style of the corporate trader. US TV soaps *Dallas*, the most popular programme in the world in 1980, and *Dynasty* (which attracted audiences of over 250 million in the first half of the decade) both revolved around fabulously wealthy oil families. They became famous for cliffhanger endings ('Who shot JR?'), outrageous villains and equally over the top styling (the official *Dynasty* website is called shoulderpads.net).

As Blake Carrington's vengeful ex-wife Alexis, Joan Collins became one of the make-up icons of the period. Bouffant hair, perfect matte foundation, dark rimmed eyes, brightly glossed lips –

such immaculate grooming hadn't been seen since the fifties when Collins first emerged from the Rank Charm School. But whereas the post-war look was above all ladylike, eighties make-up had a touch of masculine aggression. Faces were hard and sculpted – a sharp line of rouge over shaded hollow cheeks – and colours were strident. In 1983 Estée Lauder produced a range of lipsticks and nail polishes called Scandalous Scarlet, Stormy Rose and Raging Red, and a best-selling varnish from the period was Sally Hansen's 'Hard-as-Nails'. Alexis Carrington's perfectly manicured, scarlet claws were a perfect weapon for *Dynasty*'s famous catfights, and in 1983 Revlon made Joan Collins the face of their new perfume 'Scoundrel'.

Targeted at a generation of shoulder-padded executives, the signature fragrances of the eighties captured the hard-edged mood of the period, and came on strong. Giorgio Beverley Hills (1981) – the first perfume to be advertised by scented strips in magazines – was banned from restaurants because of its overpowering smell. Calvin Klein's Obsession and Dior's Poison launched in 1985, both played with ideas of sex, danger and female empowerment. Perfume and make-up were not just about attracting the opposite sex, but establishing a dominant female presence.

Superwomen

A new generation of supermodels; Claudia Schiffer, Cindy Crawford, Linda Evangelista, Naomi Campbell, and Christy Turlington, became more famous than the designers they worked for, epitomising the transition of the model from a nameless mannequin into an international celebrity and a hugely wealthy businesswoman in her own right. Linda Evangelista infamously told *Vogue* that she wouldn't get out of bed for less than $10,000 a day, a figure that came to seem almost modest by the early 1990s when Christy Turlington signed a contract with Maybelline worth a reported $800,000 for twelve days' work a year.

The ultimate 'Material Girl', Madonna epitomised this new mood of female empowerment. Arriving in New York at the age of eighteen, with only $35 in her pocket, she released her first album in 1983, and by the early 90s she had become the highest paid female recording artist of all time, and one of the most famous people in the world.

With each album Madonna created a new image, changing her hair and make-up; transforming herself from New York street urchin to Hollywood glamour queen to soft-core porn star. Girls imitated her look – bleaching the roots of their hair blonde and turning moles into beauty spots, donning fishnet tights, crucifix jewellery and short lacy tops that exposed their belly buttons. Thanks both to Madonna and to the arrival of low-cut jeans, the stomach was to become the new erogenous zone of the fin de siécle.

It wasn't just Madonna's style that attracted fans; it was her attitude. In 1985, Madonna told *Time* magazine that her childhood heroines were nuns, because they were pure and disciplined, and Hollywood film stars Carole Lombard and Marilyn Monroe, because they were so feminine and sexy. She also recalled that her favourite song was Nancy Sinatra's *These Boots Are Made for Walkin'*; 'that made one hell of an impression on me. And when she said, 'Are you ready, boots, start walkin',' it was like, yeah, give me some of those go-go boots. I want to walk on a few people.' Madonna wasn't being changed by men, or for men, she was doing it for herself.

Self-transformation was a major theme of the 1980s whether you wanted to be prime minister or a pop star or even a princess. The world watched agog as Lady Diana Spencer mutated from 'Shy Di' – a typical Sloane in minimal make-up, Laura Ashley skirt and Benetton sweater – into Princess Diana, an international icon of fashion and beauty. The Diana haircut was one of the most popular styles of the eighties, and sales of navy blue mascara and her favourite blue eyeliner boomed.

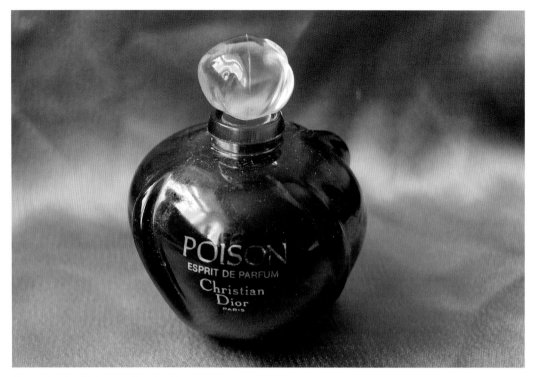

Vintage bottle of Poison perfume by Dior.

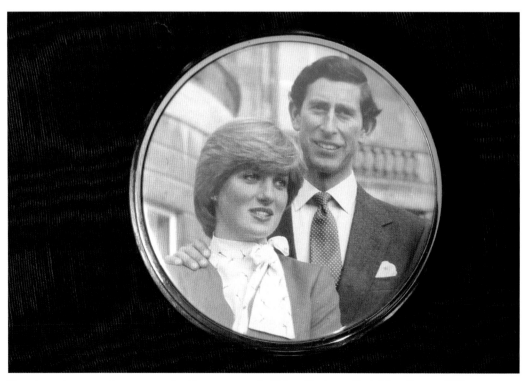

Mascot powder compact commemorating the engagement of Prince Charles and Lady Diana Spencer, 1981.

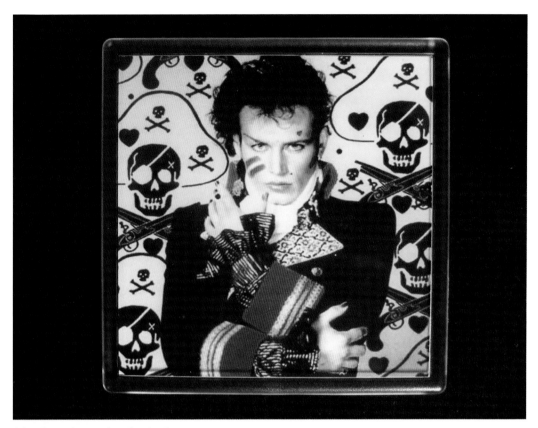

Adam Ant make-up mirror (modern).

Boys Just Want To Have Fun

Glamorous makeovers, aided by lashings of cosmetics and hair products, weren't just restricted to the girls. The most extravagant figures of the new romantic movement that burst from the English club scene at the dawn of the 'Look at me eighties' were undoubtedly the boys: Boy George (born George O'Dowd), who scaled new heights of theatrical androgyny in his Kabuki style make-up and long plaits (the popular press coined the term 'gender-bender'); Adam Ant (born Stuart Goddard), a post-modern Prince Charming in pirate gear and tribal face paint, and host of bands from Steve Strange's Visage (named after his predilection for make-up) to Birmingham's Duran Duran with their frilly shirts, big hair and black eyeliner.

The new romantics abandoned the nihilism and deliberate ugliness of punk in favour of sparkly hedonistic glamour. In the same way as East End barrow boys turned themselves into City traders, Filofax in one hand mobile phone in the other; so working-class kids from the suburbs and the provinces raided the dressing-up box, slapped on the make-up and hair gel, and reinvented themselves as the leading style-makers of the day. Regulars at Billy's in Soho and the famous Blitz club in Covent Garden (where the movement took off) included future celebrities; from pop stars – Boy George was the Blitz cloakroom attendant – to fashion designers – Stephen Jones and John Galliano – along with a sprinkling of embryo film-makers and journalists who would publicise the phenomenon in pop videos (another eighties innovation) and new magazines. *The Face* and *i-D* were both launched in 1980 and became the style and design bibles of the period.

Designer Style

Design was the religion of the eighties, and it was even granted its own temple when Terrence Conran opened the Design Museum in London in 1989. Whether you were an Armani-clad city trader or wearing a Fila tracksuit on the football terraces, label mania gripped every level of the market, and mugging people for their designer trainers emerged as a new crime. Even the most basic products were transformed into status symbols – expensive bottled mineral water appeared on the dinner table and the dressing table as the Evian Brumasiteur became a favourite facial spritz. Critics of designer water pointed out that Evian read backwards spelt naïve.

Feel the Burn

Re-designing the body was another 1980s preoccupation and there was even a new designer flab. In 1980 *Vogue* reported on the discovery of cellulite in France. Though British doctors dismissed it as 'a chic French pseudonym for fat' anxiety about bulging orange peel skin spawned a wealth of cellulite busting creams and also helped fuel the exercise craze. Gym membership and sales of home exercise equipment boomed. On British breakfast TV (also introduced in the eighties) Diana 'The Green Goddess' Moran and 'Mad' Lizzie Webb roused the nation with morning exercises and if their routines didn't wake you up, then the sight of their day-glo gym kits and bright make-up certainly would.

Fashionable fitness crazes included 'dancercise' and aerobics – a system of exercise originally devised in 1968 by Dr Kenneth H. Cooper, a physician at the San Antonio Air Force Hospital in Texas. Popularised by Jane Fonda's Workout Videos, which sold a staggering 17 million copies and topped the Billboard charts in the mid-eighties, the number of aerobics participants in the US swelled from an estimated 6 million in 1978 to 22 million in 1987. 'Feel the Burn' became one of the catchphrases of the decade – a symbol of the go-getting eighties attitude – and even if you remained a couch potato (sitting down to watch your exercise on TV with a packet of Hob Nobs) leg warmers, head bands, footless tights and the infamous shell suit became must have fashion wear.

Calorie Counting

With stretchy Lycra revealing every bump and lump, dieting flourished along with exercise. Audrey Eyton's F-Plan diet was the international publishing sensation of 1982 – the F standing for fibre but also leading to flatulence as dieters masticated their way through pulses and vegetables. As millions slimmed (or at least bought the books), the diet industry got fat. In 1988 Americans spent $33 million on diet related products, but that same year sixty-seven deaths were reported in the US from anorexia nervosa. Along with calorie and cholesterol control came a new concern about eating disorders. Bulimia nervosa was first identified as a psychiatric illness in 1979; surveys carried out in the 1980s revealed that growing numbers of teenagers considered themselves overweight and were unhappy about their body image. In 1983 the singer Karen Carpenter died from anorexia-related complications and in the confessional nineties many eighties celebrities from Jane Fonda to Princess Diana admitted to having suffered from eating disorders.

Protect and Survive

As the 1980s drew to a close looking after the body became increasingly important and, after an age of excess, self-denial became fashionable. Growing awareness of cancer and heart disease caused many to give up sunbathing and smoking. With the arrival of the Aids epidemic leading a healthy life became a matter of increasing concern and women were encouraged to take

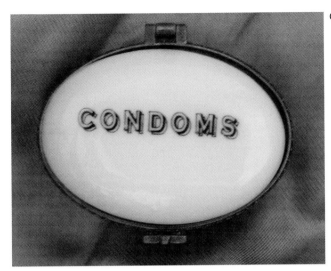

Ceramic box for condoms.

responsibility for themselves in the bedroom, as they had done in the boardroom. The must-have handbag accessory at the end of the decade was not a lipstick or a sparkly compact but a packet of condoms.

On the eighties dressing table

Label mania and glitz affected cosmetics as much as fashion. Chanel's make-up containers were emblazoned with a prominent CC logo; Dior advertised its lipsticks as 'couture clad' in blue and gold; YSL lipsticks came in shiny gold cases. At the other end of the market Avon captured the jocular spirit of post-modernism, producing flavoured lipgloss in novelty plastic containers shaped like ice creams and children's crayons.

Though a small number of metal compacts were produced typically these were for the luxury and gift market. Disposable plastics remained the favourite medium and increasingly women were buying cosmetics from high street chemists rather than exclusive department stores. In Britain the number of Superdrug stores mushroomed from seventy-seven in 1979 to 650 in 1990 and Boots was a favourite venue for affordable beauty products.

Mass market make-up boomed and in an economic climate dominated by big business takeovers individual companies were gobbled up by major corporations: Elizabeth Arden was purchased by Unilever; Helena Rubinstein was taken over by L'Oréal; and Vidal Sassoon sold his name to Procter and Gamble.

With the fashion for big hair, hair products became increasingly big business. Mousses, gels and volumisers were must have items for boys as well as girls. Sun-In hair lightener provided affordable blonde highlights, whether you wanted to look like David Sylvian, Madonna, or maybe even Kermit the Frog (if as sometimes happened highlights went not blonde but green). Interest in celebrity hairstyles made hairdressers famous. John Frieda (whose clients included Lady Diana Spencer) developed his own line of shampoos in the mid-eighties and professional hair care products bearing the name of a famous stylist would become an industry standard.

Indoor tanning units were a popular craze and one of America's fastest growing industries. However with growing fears of skin cancer (incidences of malignant melanoma increased by 500% from 1950-85) by the end of the eighties sun tanning was condemned as dangerous and fake tan flourished.

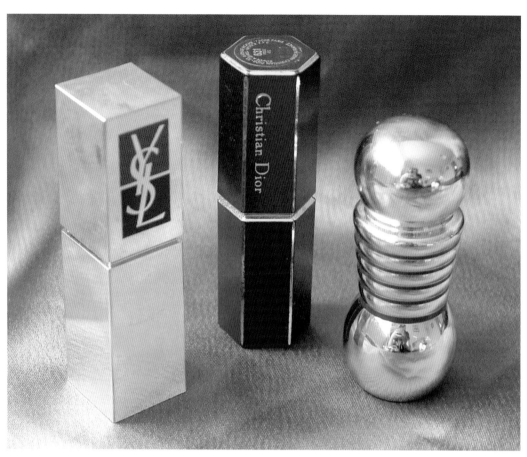

Classic designer lipsticks by YSL and Dior.

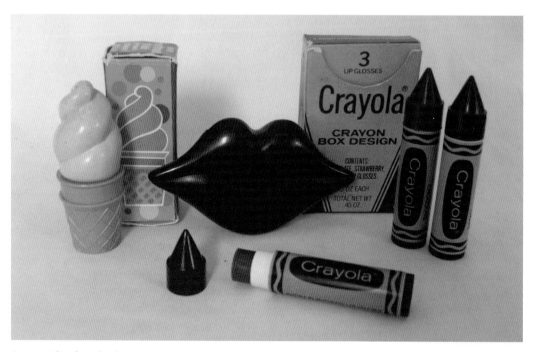

Avon novelty plastic lipgloss containers, 1980s.

Skincare was the other big story of the period. Reflecting the fact that the baby boom generation was getting older, moisturisers were now described as 'anti-ageing creams', fighting wrinkles with mysterious ingredients (liposomes, Retin A, polyenergisers) and fulsome promises. 'The ideal modern cosmetics consumer would be a biochemist married to a philologist,' observed *Vogue* in 1987. 'One of them could work out what the product actually does to the skin, while the other tried to make sense of the claims.'

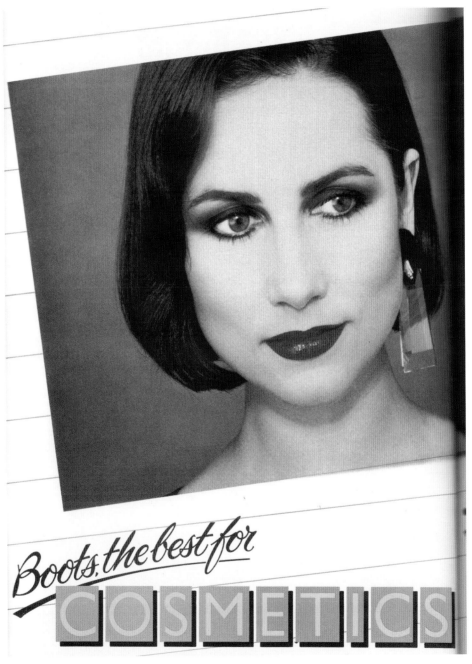

Advertisement for Boots Cosmetics 1983.

CHAPTER TWELVE

Bling, Botox or the Burqa?

Beauty at the Dawn of the New Millenium

I N 1990 MARGARET Thatcher resigned as Prime Minister and the Victoria and Albert Museum in London asked visitors to donate their shoulder pads to make a sculpture commemorating the 1980s. *Vogue*'s first cover of the new decade featured a handful of supermodels and a question 'The 1990s – What next?'

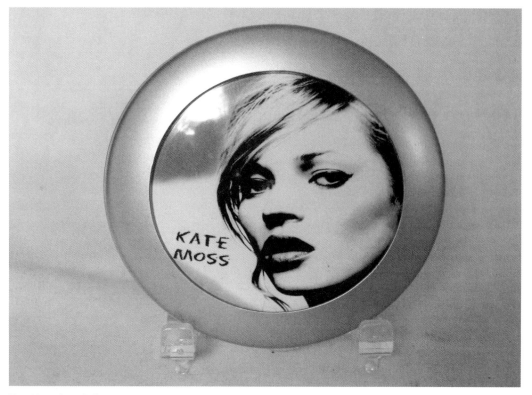

Kate Moss plastic light-up compact mirror, 2008.

There wasn't a simple answer. The turn of the Twentieth Century was characterised not by a single unifying look but a plethora of multicultural styles spread by music, celebrities, an expanding media and perhaps most significantly by the internet, which became the favourite source of information, entertainment and shopping across the world.

Grunge and Heroine Chic

As the confident eighties gave way to the anxious nineties, yuppie dress and power make-up fell from grace and a new 'anti-fashion' was grunge.

Inspired by grunge music (exemplified by the distorted guitars and angst ridden lyrics of Seattle-based band Nirvana) and embodied by British supermodel Kate Moss, grunge style was emaciated, wasted and coolly unkempt. Nirvana's 1991 breakthrough single might have been called *Smells like Teen Spirit,* a US deodorant and hair care range, but grunge wasn't big on personal hygiene.

Clothes were muted in colour with a thrift shop feel: jeans, plaid shirts, down at heel boots. Long hair (preferably not too clean or too brushed) was worn by both girls and boys. Make-up looked as though you'd either forgotten to put it on (the 'no make-up' make-up look) or hadn't remembered to take it off: lots of thick black eyeliner (make it 'ragged and rough, as though you have slept in it' advised an online grunge make-up guide); nude-coloured lips and a pale foundation with no blusher and certainly no bronzer. The only reason for dedicated grunge addicts to go outdoors would be to visit a rock festival, the off-licence or their dealer.

Dubbed 'Heroin Chic' the grunge look which appeared in magazines and advertising campaigns attracted some heavyweight criticism in the early nineties. 'Fashion photos in the last few years have made heroin addiction seem glamorous and sexy and cool,' objected President Clinton. 'And as some of those people in those images start to die now, it has become obvious that that is not true, you do not need to glamorize addiction to sell clothes.' Heroin might not have been cool, but as long as you retained your fashion edge, a partying lifestyle apparently was. In 2005 Moss was dubbed 'Cocaine Kate' by the tabloid press, when the *Daily Mirror* published pictures that appeared to show her snorting class A drugs. After a police investigation, and an initial panic when she lost several advertising contracts, Moss went from strength to strength, producing her own clothing range for Top Shop and remaining the face of Rimmel: 'Kate Moss is a worldwide inspiration and leader in fashion and beauty, and has been an iconic face for Rimmel London,' enthused Stephen Mormoris, Senior Vice President of Coty Beauty. 'I am thrilled we are continuing our professional partnership, and that she will be an inspiration for the Rimmel consumer as our official ambassador.'

Subcultural styles – Tats and Piercings

Drug-related or not, youth and underground subcultures had an ever more significant impact on beauty at the turn of the century. The most obvious was the vogue for tattooing and piercing – traditionally a male preserve and the mark of clearly delineated or outsider groups in the West (sailors, prisoners, the fetish scene) – which emerged from the 1990s as unisex decorations, sported by everybody from celebrities downwards. Tattoo parlours flourished on the high street; a BBC survey of 10 to 15-year-olds in 2003 revealed that one in four children had a family member with at least one 'tat' or piercing; school girls flaunted their belly button rings and damaged their tooth enamel with tongue bars.

'Body Art or Tramp Stamp?' demanded the media as women as well as men decorated their bodies with a cultural cocktail of images ranging from Celtic strapwork to Japanese characters. Some amusement was created in the press when it was revealed that football superstar David Beckham (whose famously beautiful body was covered with 'pick-and-mix' tattoos in Latin, Hebrew and Chinese) had misspelt his wife Victoria's name in Hindi on his forearm.

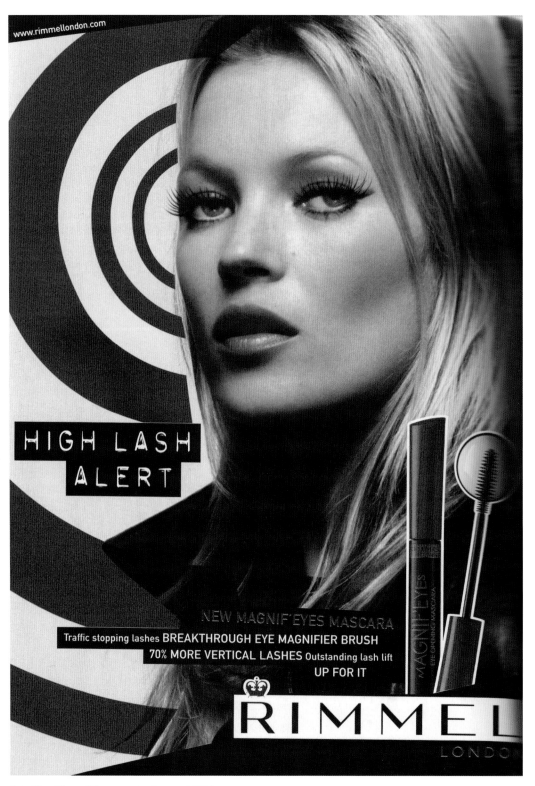

Kate Moss Rimmel Mascara advertisement, 2006.

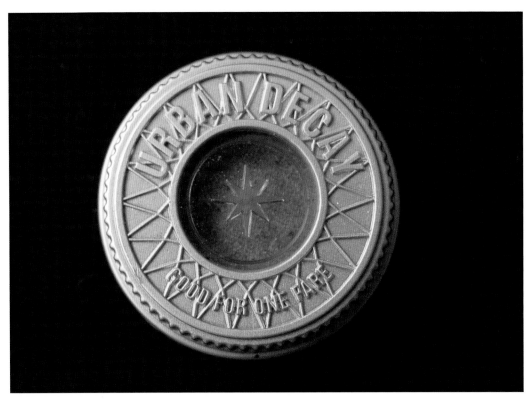

Urban decay eye shadow in the shape of a New York subway token.

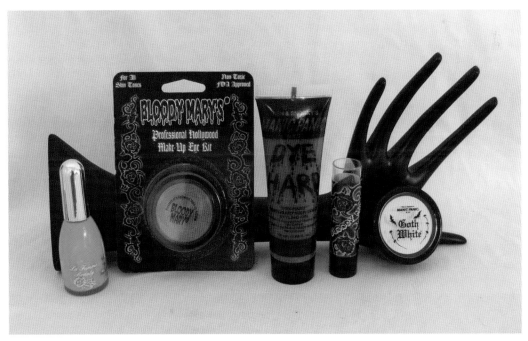

Goth make-up selection: La Femme Beauty fluorescent green nail varnish; Bloody Mary's Eye shadow; Manic Panic Dye Hard Hair Colour; Bloody Mary's Blood Lipstick; Manic Panic Goth White powder compact.

But even if you couldn't actually read them, your tattoos would provide a lasting reminder of attitudes to beauty and the body at the dawn of the Twenty-first Century. This was a period overwhelmed with a global supermarket of products and there were innumerable looks to choose from.

Goth

Goth, which emerged as an offshoot of punk in the late seventies, became increasingly popular from the nineties providing an ideal uniform for teenage alienation, and offering a dramatic alternative to digitally enhanced pictures of mainstream beauty. You didn't need to be a size zero to look good as a Goth and corpse make-up was the perfect concealer for adolescent acne. Cosmetics and clothes were inspired by a range of influences, from gothic novels to horror films: favourite colours included red, purple, lime green and above all black.

Goth along with emo, heavy metal and cyber-punk related styles, helped inspire the creation of new beauty brands. Bloody Mary, launched in 2000 by Hollywood special effects make-up artist Bobbie Weiner, offered a wide range of Goth cosmetics including Pale Death foundation, Blood Red mascara and Black Blood lipstick. In 1995, when she couldn't find the right shade of purple nail polish, Sandy Lerner started the cosmetics company Urban Decay. The name was a deliberate attempt to avoid the fluffy and feminine associations of make-up and advertisements had the tag line 'Does pink make you puke?' Eye shadows (the company's best-selling product) came packaged in a grey plastic compact shaped like a New York subway token and with shades called Smog, Uzi, Roach and Acid Rain, Urban Decay took street style inside the department store.

Bling Bling

Hip hop, originating in the 1980s with African American and Latino youth in the New York Bronx, was another movement which made the transition from urban underground to mainstream fashion; as kids across the world adopted rap music, slang and styles. One of the most ubiquitous 'gangsta' trends was 'sagging' trousers (deriving from the prison custom of removing belts so that inmates couldn't hang themselves) and which made boys waddle like penguins, giving onlookers plenty of time to check out their designer underwear. Expensive labels and logos were an essential part of the rapper look and 'bling bling' was expressed not just in big jewellery but cosmetic accessories. The ultimate rapper purchase was a mouthful of gold teeth covers or 'grillz'. 'More gangsta than any accessory on the market, GRILLZ are more than just Gold Teeth, they help all your homies know that you are the ultimate pimp. All the ladies will want to see your grill!' promised one contemporary advertisement.

Whilst 'homies' enhanced their teeth, for the ladies (aka 'biatches') there were hair extensions and nail extensions. Modern acrylic nails had been developed in the late 1970s by American dentist Dr Stuart Nordstrom after a patient (a female manicurist) remarked that the material used to prepare temporary tooth caps smelt like false nails, which she complained were not very good. Dr Nordstrom set to work and came up with SolarNail Liquid – described by his company Creative Nail Design as the first-ever monomer formulation for greater nail strength and flexibility and the first product to deliver a natural, non-yellowing nail colour.

Better, more affordable artificial nails and the street fashion for digital bling revolutionised the industry. Manicurists became 'nail technicians' and according to American industry bible *Nails Magazine*, in the US alone their number rose from around 80,000 in 1982 to 175,832 in 1993, more than doubling in a decade. Nail painting became 'nail art' and huge talons were decorated with elaborate airbrushed pictures, stick-on rhinestones, and dangling nail charms suspended from drilled holes. Whereas ladies in the 1930s had shown off their elegant manicured fingers playing with compacts and cigarette cases, the ultimate way of demonstrating acrylic nails was texting on the mobile.

Make-up too went bling. You could decorate your eyelids with Hard Candy 'Bling Bling' Glitter Eye shadow and your eyelashes with tiny stick on gems. Dior's Princess Ring – a huge, mirrored rapper style ring edged with diamante – opened up to reveal eye and lip colours. In the US, Haute Couture Beauty produced mascara in a Swarovski case selling for $589; which might well have seemed like the most expensive make-up in the world until 2006, when for her twenty-fifth birthday a Las Vegas client commissioned a version in solid 18-carat gold studded with real blue and pink diamonds, which complete with a matching jewelled lipstick cost a reported $14 million.

Even Barbie became 'ghetto fabulous'. Fighting competition from the trendy Bratz Dolls, Mattel launched 'Bling Bling Barbie' in 2005. Targeted at girls aged six plus, Barbie came complete with stiletto-heeled silver boots, micro-miniskirt, belly-bar, protruding nipples and a handbag for her mini make-up and mobile. Her outfit hovered between street style and streetwalker and her face was transformed with multi-coloured glitter eyeshadow, heavily mascara'd extended eyelashes and Angelina Jolie-style swollen lips.

Come to the Botox Party

It wasn't just Barbie who was getting a 'trout pout'. The turn of the century saw the rise of cosmetic surgery, transformed from a secret shame (advertised in discreet small ads) into a multi-billion dollar global business, promoted in dedicated magazines, demonstrated in makeover television programmes, and endorsed implicitly and explicitly by celebrities who accessorised skinny bodies with gi-normous breasts and flaunted wrinkle-free faces whatever their age. 'Oh, sweetie, one more facelift on this one and she'll have a beard,' commented *Absolutely Fabulous'* Patsy happily as she leafed through the gossip magazines.

Figures from the International Society of Aesthetic Plastic Surgery revealed that the top three countries for cosmetic operations in 2000 were the US (143,676), followed by Brazil (66,090) then the UK (24, 336). By 2006 spending on cosmetic procedures, both surgical and non-surgical, had reached nearly £500m in Britain (four times more than in 2001), and market analysts Datamonitor predicted this would treble to £1.476bn by 2011.

As consumption of nip and tuck went up, so the age range went down. Whereas in the Twentieth Century plastic surgery was most typically associated with the over fifties, in the new millennium, there was a new target audience. The American Society for Aesthetic Plastic Surgery (ASAPS) recorded 11.7 million surgical and non-surgical cosmetic procedures performed in the United States in 2007. People aged 35–50 had the most, with forty-six per cent of the total. The 51–64 age group came next with only twenty-five per cent of the market; and snapping at the heels of the Botox-ed, liposuction-ed and microdermabraded bodies of the older generations were those aged 19–34 with a twenty-one per cent share, and a particular fondness for breast augmentation. Even teenagers too young to go into a bar in the US were old enough for a bit of chemical rejuvenation. According to the *New York Post* by May 2008, the latest must-have purchase for girls going to their high school prom was not just the perfect dress but an injection of collagen in the lips and a shot of Botox between the eyes.

Irrespective of age, Botox was by far the most popular treatment in the States (as across the world) with 3,181, 592 procedures carried out in 2007. Botox was affordable (the average price of a half-hour session was $380 (£190)), readily available and quick – you could get your wrinkles injected in your lunch hour and still have time for a sandwich. The development of non-surgical 'less-invasive' techniques fuelled the cosmetic industry boom but anxieties were expressed about the long-term effects of a quick fix. 'Does Botox get into the brain?' asked *Newsweek* in 2008, reporting on new research revealing that when rats were injected with Botox, the toxin migrated from the whisker muscles to the brainstem, where it disrupted neuronal activity.

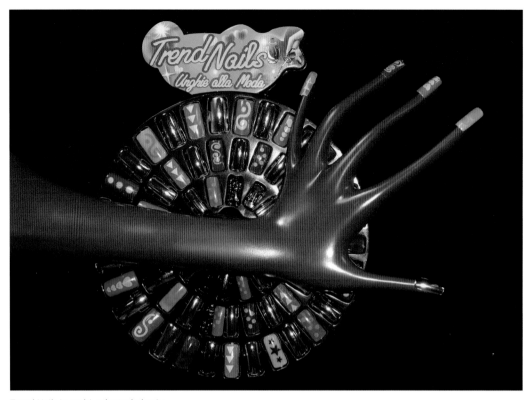

Trend Nails in multi-coloured plastic.

Dior Princess Ring, eyeshadow compact.

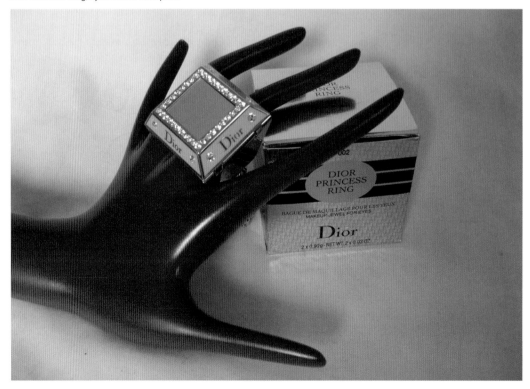

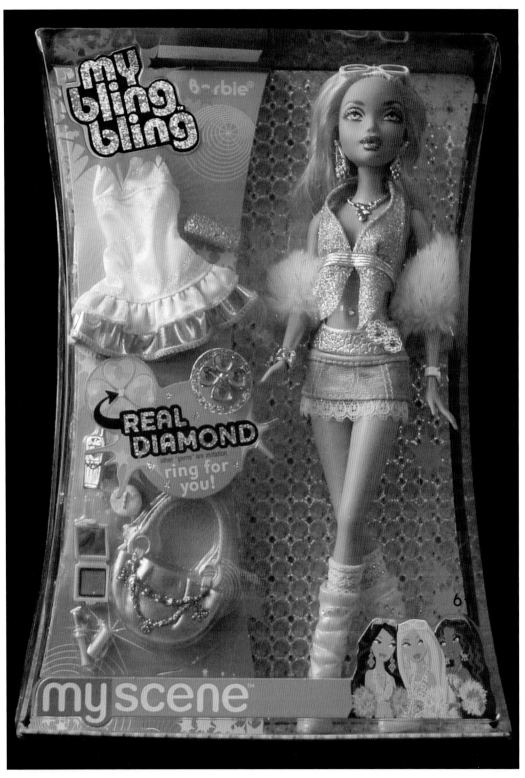

My Bling Bling Barbie, Mattel, 2005.

And as far as critics were concerned, it was madness to consider it anyway. Numerous deaths and hospitalisations from cosmetic surgery were reported in the late nineties/early noughties. Celebrity victims; Lesley 'Trout Pout' Ash, the British actress whose collagen lip implants went tragically wrong, and American socialite Jocelyn Wildenstein who spent a rumoured $2 million remodelling her face and body only to be dubbed 'the Bride of Wildenstein' both demonstrated in the remorseless glare of publicity what could happen when intervention went wrong. Increasing concerns were expressed about the physical safety of procedures, the training of practitioners (in Britain no medical qualifications were required to inject patients with fillers), and the psychology of a society prepared to go to any lengths to maintain a perceived ideal of youth and beauty. One of the ironies of the period is that while Muslim women were feared, pitied and stigmatised for covering their faces with the veil, growing numbers of women in the West were happy to submit to the knife, the laser, and to inject their skin with a product derived from one of the most poisonous naturally occurring substances in the world – both attitudes to the female body arguably representing a certain extremism.

Age-Defying Creams – Holding Back the Years

In a culture obsessed with youth but dominated by an ageing population, beauty was hard work. Women from Madonna to Sharon Osbourne to Joan Collins showed that you could preserve your iconic status into middle and even pensionable age; but only if you were prepared to expend Herculean amounts of effort and money on exercise; cosmetic surgery and make-up. 'Whatever happened to ageing gracefully?' asked Miranda in *Sex and the City*. 'It got old,' replied Carrie.

For those who didn't want to resort to Botox or the burqa, creams became increasingly important. Anti-ageing, anti-wrinkle, lifting, firming, radiant, and time-delay were principle buzzwords in skincare. In the US the value of the anti-ageing skincare market grew sixty-three per cent between 2002–07 to $1.6billion, and demand boomed everywhere from the supermarket to the prestige department store. In 2005 Forbes.com produced a list of the fourteen most expensive products they could find, beginning in terms of price with Estée Lauder's Re Nutriv eye cream ($100 per oz) which by the time they got to RéVive Intensité Volumizing Serum, at $600 per ounce, began to seem like a bit of a bargain. But it wasn't just high-prices that were plumping the value of the market like a pair of collagen implanted lips; it was high volume. Whereas in the past women had made do with a single pot of cold cream, now just to moisturise the face alone there was a dressing table full of beauty basics – separate moisturisers for day and night; different creams for summer and winter; specialist serums to go underneath the moisturisers; dedicated eye and lip creams to go on top. And that's to say nothing of cleansers, toners, exfoliators, reviving masks and make-up. Cosmetic companies might have stressed their green credentials with recyclable containers and eco-friendly contents – but no one was going to encourage consumers to consume less. Even if you only went into a shop for a single product; special offers, three for the price of two, free gifts, and loyalty points would invariably seduce you to buy more.

Professional Beauty

With so much to choose from expert advice was sought after. TV makeover programmes showed how with the help of bullying beauty gurus, ugly ducklings could be turned into swans. Women's magazines and internet beauty sites offered in-depth advice on products and technique; Stila even produced a talking eyeshadow compact that gave a step-by-step application guide at the press of a button. Like Stila many of the most prestigious brands of the day; Shu Uemura, Nars, M.A.C, Ruby & Millie, and Bobbi Brown, were started by professional make-up artists and packaging expressed this provenance.

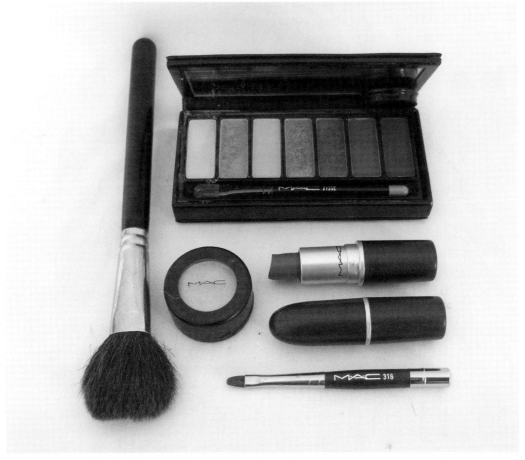

M.A.C cosmetics and brushes. The professional look of modern make-up.

In the same way that turn of the century kitchen appliances came in brushed steel rather than traditional domestic white, mirroring the working environment of the professional TV chef; so make-up by companies such as M.A.C and Nars was contained not in shiny gilt compacts, but in sleek and minimalist black containers. The understated packaging offered consumers a sense of professional expertise and beauty by association with celebrity stylists. This was sophisticated make-up, and in an increasingly visual and high-tech age looking good had never been more important.

Camera Face

In the 1920s and 30s the arrival of the affordable domestic camera had made women more conscious of their appearance. By the dawn of the new millennium everybody had a camera on their phone; at the press of a button a photo could be instantly sent to all your contacts; and thanks to the internet (MySpace, FaceBook, etc.) personal snaps could be publicised around the world.

For celebrities, the most photographed people on the planet, digital photography was both a blessing and a curse. In publicity pictures and a controlled environment photo shop and digital enhancement could make them more beautiful than ever before. But once you'd courted the

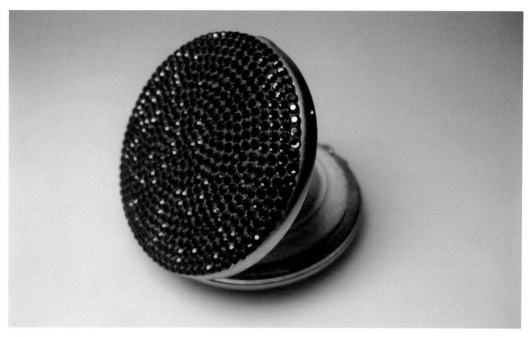

Judith Leiber compact decorated with red rhinestones. *Gray's Antiques Market*

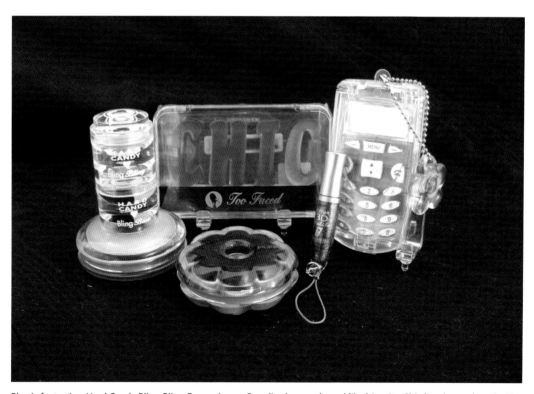

Plastic fantastic – Hard Candy Bling Bling Eye make-up; Pura lipgloss packaged like biscuits; Chic lip gloss palette by Too Faced; plastic lip gloss palette in the form of a mobile phone (made in China); Bourjois Mini Effect 3D Mobile Lipgloss, designed to be attached to a mobile phone.

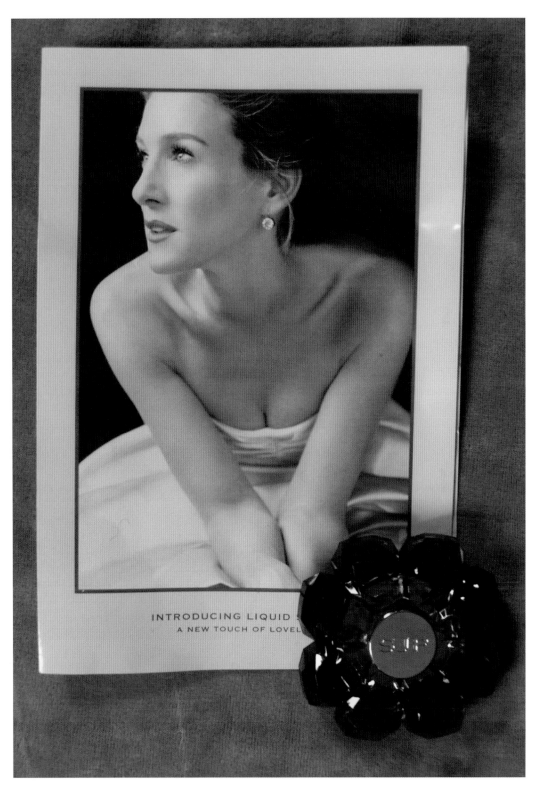

INTRODUCING LIQUID
A NEW TOUCH OF LOVEL

SJP compact mirror, part of the Sarah Jessica Parker fragrance range.

press the gloves were off. A new genre of celebrity magazine emerged at the turn of the century: *OK, Heat, Closer* – the bitchy younger sisters of *Hello* – whose aim was to expose (often literally) the soft white underbelly of stardom. Paparazzi zoned in on the wobbly thigh, the unshaven armpit, the age-knotted hand, and the tell-tale surgery scars. For the first time since the development of photography the pictures everyone wanted were the ones that showed the worst, and women weren't the only victims.

Make-up for Men

Tabloid photographers focused their lenses on male wrinkles, celebrity bald spots and beer bellies – a new word 'moob' (short for man boob) appeared in online dictionaries. Men too were increasingly subject to criticism and worried about how they looked and what they were expected to be. With growing equality between the sexes, women took them on in the boardroom and gave as good as they got in the bedroom. 'You have a lot of nerve telling me to get a wax. If you were in Aruba the natives could bead your back. And it's not just there: every time I blow you I feel like I'm flossing,' *Sex and the City*'s Samantha told one of her many partners.

With the rise of strong, successful and independent women came different male archetypes; the 'new man', 'metrosexual man', and 'the toy boy'. Footballers burst into tears on the pitch when they missed a goal and played with their hair like girls: the most macho men were vulnerable to physical insecurity. Former British Deputy Prime Minister John Prescott admitted to suffering from bulimia. 'Smooth operator: Has TV chef Gordon Ramsay had Botox?' asked the *Daily Mail* hopefully in May 2008, and even Homer Simpson had liposuction.

The number of men resorting to cosmetic treatment increased by an astonishing 886% between 1997-2007. Botox and laser hair removal were the favourite non-surgical procedures; liposuction, breast reduction and hair transplants appeared in the top five operations. Demand for male grooming products flourished. Market analysts Mintel reported that UK sales were worth £685 million in 2004, projecting a rise to £821 million by 2009. 'That's £136 millions of added insecurity,' moaned *Observer* journalist Will Leith, reporting on the launch of Clinique's M Cover, a new concealer for men. ' As well as worrying about the closeness of our shave, the look and colour of our hair and how we smell, we will also be paranoid about the fact that our complexions are not flawless … Concealer is about pretence. It's about wanting to look unworn, untested, smooth and blameless.'

Sisters are doing it for themselves

At the dawn of the Twenty-first Century, as men agonised like Victorian virgins on their wedding night about changing notions of masculinity and the fact that their sponge bags were turning into make-up bags, women embraced the confusion and the possibilities of the modern age. The pressure to keep young and beautiful was perhaps more intense than ever and the methods used to achieve this goal were just as time consuming, painful and potentially dangerous as they ever had been in the past. But women themselves were very different from their ladylike Victorian ancestors.

The fin de siecle saw the emergence of a new female archetype: the 30-something singleton epitomised in Britain by Helen Fielding's *Bridget Jones* in her big pants, and in the US by Carrie, Miranda, Charlotte, and Samantha (in her pearl thong); the single girls of HBO's hugely successful TV series *Sex and the City* (1998–2004). As they searched New York for sex, love and designer shoes, the heroines submitted themselves to every modern-day beauty fad from chemical peels to Brazilian waxing. Some accused the show of betraying feminism with its portrayal of women as sex and shopping obsessed fashionistas on an endless quest for the ideal boyfriend but *Sex and the City* claimed its own feminist agenda. These were strong, modern women who, sustained by friendship and a sense of humour, made their own choices and mistakes. Their pursuit of fashion and beauty was not for the sake of men, but to make themselves look and feel fabulous with or without a partner. 'The show is a valentine to being single ...' claimed Kim Cattrall. 'Being single used to mean that nobody wanted you; now it means you're pretty sexy and you're taking your time deciding how you want your life to be ... and who you want to spend it with.'

And what you wanted to look like. For Western women in the Twenty-first century, whether you were a ladette, a lipstick lesbian or a yummy mummy; whether you opted to tattoo your thigh or Botox your face; whether you invested fortunes on designer creams and cosmetics or decided to throw them away and let nature take its inevitable course; what you did to your face and body was up to you.

On the Twenty-first Century Dressing Table

Famous designer brands flourished in the age of bling. Must-have products ranged from long-established products such as Elizabeth Arden's 8-hour cream and Chanel lipstick; to new handbag essentials, YSL Touche Éclat (1992) designed to hide bags under the eyes, and Lancôme Juicy Tubes lip glosses (2000). Collagen enhanced lip plumpers were another new favourite, designed to plump the lips without recourse to surgery.

Maybelline mascara remained the world's best-known and best-selling mascara (one is allegedly sold every 1.9 seconds) and in 2008 Estée Lauder and Lancôme both launched rival battery operated mascaras. Competition to create beautiful eyes was fierce and not always honourable. Both L'Oréal and Rimmel were found guilty by the Advertising Standards Authority of misleading the public in their mascara advertisements and neglecting to mention that their respective stars, Penelope Cruz and Kate Moss, appeared to have received some lash fluttering assistance from either false eyelashes or digital enhancement.

Photoshopped or not, models and actresses were a major influence on beauty. In 1994 the Sudanese supermodel Iman (wife of David Bowie) launched her own line of prestige skincare and make-up for women of colour. Celebrities increasingly endorsed cosmetic and fragrance lines and, though the thought of what Britney Spears might smell like after her much-publicised meltdown was not automatically appealing, in 2008 Britney perfume was the leading celebrity brand in the UK with sales worth £13 million.

Make-up by make-up artists (M.A.C, Bobbi Brown, Nars, Jemma Kidd etc.) allowed ordinary women to feel like celebrities. Though packaging and increased use of professional techniques (i.e. make-up brushes) emphasised a serious, professional approach names expressed a sense of fun and new attitudes to sexuality. Nars best-selling blusher colour was 'Orgasm' – described as peachy pink with shimmer. Funky new cosmetic companies such as Hard Candy (1995) and Too Faced (est.1998) reflected the fashion for quirky glamour. Retro styling was another trend with fashionable brands such as Benefit (launched 1990) drawing on thirties Hollywood glamour and fifties fashions in compacts and packaging.

As street style came to the fore, handbag mirrors were decorated with photographs of fashionable celebrities and the mobile phone was a new target for make-up, with stick on mirrors and dangling lipstick charms.

The decorative powder compact enjoyed a limited revival, particularly in the luxury market. British accessories designer Lulu Guinness produced cosmetic containers to go with her retro inspired handbags. American purse designer Judith Leiber created colourful compacts encrusted with rhinestones. Big name companies from Dior to YSL launched limited edition compacts in various forms to match the season's new cosmetic lines, often heavily emblazoned with look-at-me logos. Reflecting interest in vintage make-up accessories, firms created compacts for the burgeoning modern 'collectables' market and Estée Lauder compacts for solid perfume and cosmetics attracted an enthusiastic following.

In the caring nineties there was also a serious side to make-up. Cosmetic companies joined in the fight against HIV and cancer. In 1992 Estée Lauder started their annual Breast Cancer Awareness Campaign and launched the pink ribbon as a worldwide symbol of breast health. Two years later M.A.C introduced their highly successful Viva Glam Lipstick 'an out spoken deep red', promoted by drag artist RuPaul, with profits going to the M.A.C AIDS Fund.

Saving the planet and green awareness were major themes. Beauty Without Cruelty promoted vegetarian beauty products made without animal testing. Firms such as Origins (est.1990) promoted organic creams and cosmetics in eco-friendly containers. However the popularity of additional skin care items such as serums and disposable cleansing wipes helped ensure that people were using and throwing away more than ever before.

If you couldn't always be green, you could be brown all year round thanks to St Tropez fake tan (launched 1996). With growing fears about skin cancer the spray tanning unit took over from sunbeds and real sunshine. Bronzing creams and tinted moisturisers became a dressing table favourite and not just with women.

According to a Boots survey, nine out of ten men thought that cosmetics and clothes could give them more pulling power than a car. In January 2008 Boots launched their No. 7 range for men including tanning and anti-ageing creams; the 'protect and perfect' formula exactly the same as that used in their female range but packaged in 'man-friendly' pale brown containers.

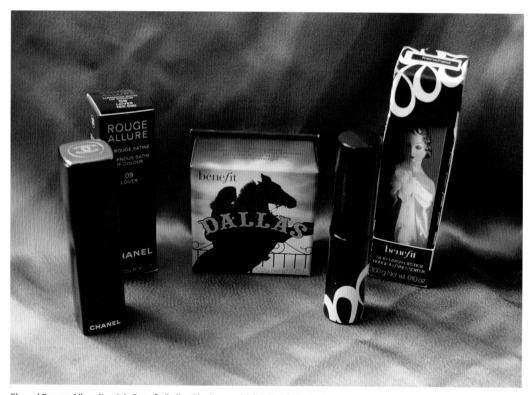

Chanel Rouge Allure lipstick; Benefit Dallas Blusher and Silky Finish Lipstick.

Buying Beauty

Collecting Compacts and Cosmetics

THIS BOOK IS predominantly illustrated with pieces from my own private collection. One of the joys of collecting cosmetic accessories is that they encompass a wide range of objects and media, from elegant powder compacts to humble deodorant tins, from Victorian silverware, to modern plastics. Some subjects are well-established collectables, others less so. A 1930s lady

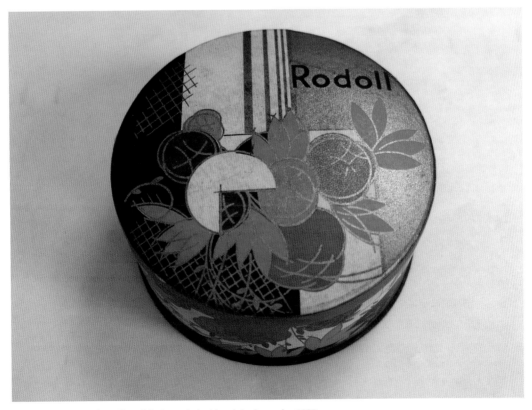

Rodoll powder box, by P.Giraud, Paris, sealed with original powder, 1930s.

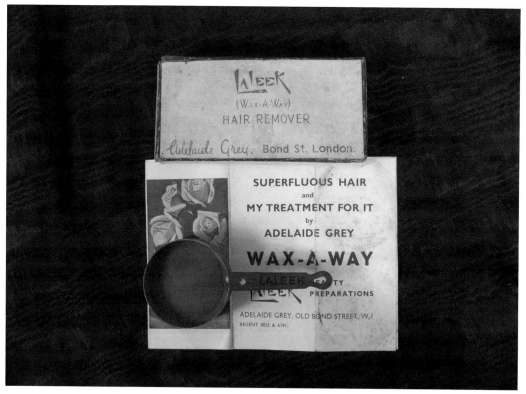

The Laleek Wax-a-Way Hair Remover by Adelaide Grey, Bond Street London, c.1940. The perfect example of a random eBay purchase and surprisingly affordable precisely because it has a very niche market.

shave or a pair of 1960s false eyelashes might not be as valuable or attractive as a fine art deco vanity case but for me they are just as representative of their times and what women did to their bodies. Paradoxically, it is often the more mundane items that are hardest to track down, both because few people bothered to keep them in the first place, and admittedly not that many want to buy them today!

Collecting advice in specific areas is included below, but some tips apply equally to every subject. Antiques-related TV programmes and newspaper articles often tend to focus on value, but as most enthusiasts know collecting is above all about passion (some unkind members of my family also refer to it as madness). Whatever your chosen area, the most important advice is to buy what you like and what stimulates your eye and brain.

Condition is a major factor and when possible it is always a good idea to purchase the best and most complete example that you can afford. Sometimes however you will have to compromise and buy something in what vendors often euphemistically describe as 'condition commensurate with age'. Seriously damaged pieces should be avoided, but rarities should not be overlooked because of a little wear and tear. Though value might be affected, it doesn't make the object any less interesting in historical terms and it also means that there can be less anxiety involved in displaying or even using it.

In forming my own collection, I have bought everywhere from antique markets to car boot fairs. A small number of dealers specialise in beauty-related items – most typically compacts and perfume bottles. Vintage fashion fairs are a good venue for cosmetic material as are dealers

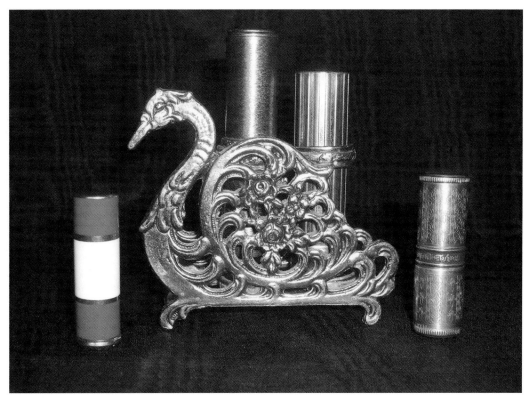

Brass lipstick caddy in the form of a swan, c.1950s/60s with a selection of vintage lipsticks.

in advertising and packaging. eBay is a useful source but caution is always necessary when you are bidding for something you can't see or touch. Check the vendor's feedback, examine descriptions and photographs carefully, and if you are not happy with an item; send it back! Having said that, eBay is wonderful for finding more unusual pieces from vintage mascaras to flapper curling tongs; you can shop across the world at the press of a button and if you know what you want, ultimately you'll probably come across it.

The more you learn, the better you will buy and the more you will appreciate your collection. Consult reference books, and the internet is a boon for checking prices, making contacts and tracking down information. Nothing however beats seeing as many objects in the flesh as you possibly can. Visit antique fairs, talk to dealers and fellow enthusiasts and if there is one join a collectors' club. Though cosmetics are not a typical museum subject, fashion galleries will sometimes include related material as will collections devoted to advertising and packaging or popular culture.

Collecting is a learning curve and above all it's fun. Hunting down objects is exciting and you never know what you will discover and whom you will meet. Owning them is also a pleasure. Some enthusiasts keep their treasures carefully packed away in acid free tissue to protect them from light and damage, but as far as I am concerned if you can't see your collection, and share it with your friends, what's the point? The main thrust of my own 'passion' is everyday beauty accessories used by women of the past, and I display them on the shelves of my study, where they can be can be enjoyed, everyday, by a woman of the present.

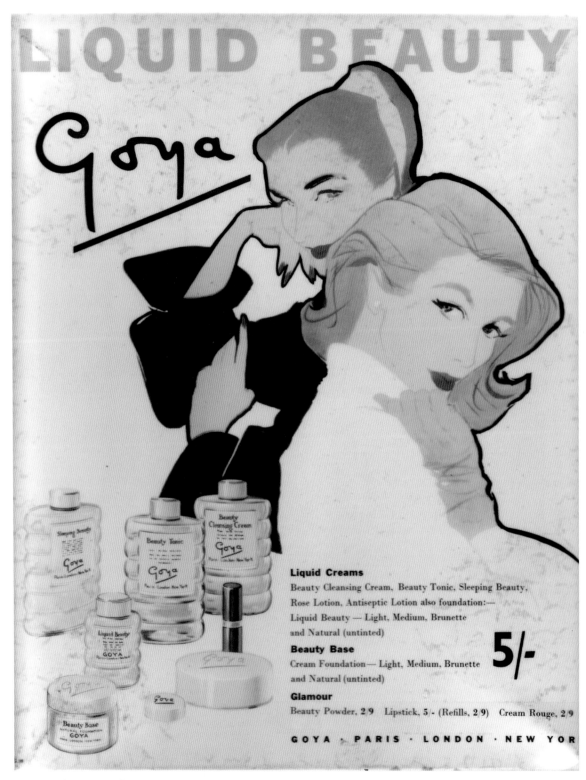

Goya Liquid Beauty tin advertising sign, 1950s.

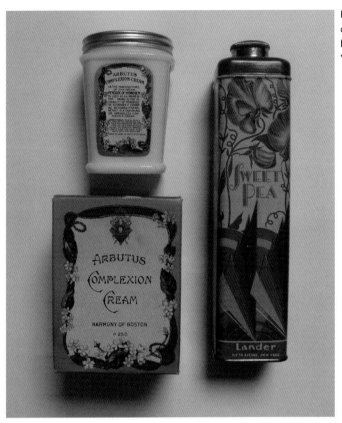

Perfect packaging: Arbutus Complexion cream by Harmony of Boston, mint and boxed; Sweet Pea talk tin by Lander, New York.

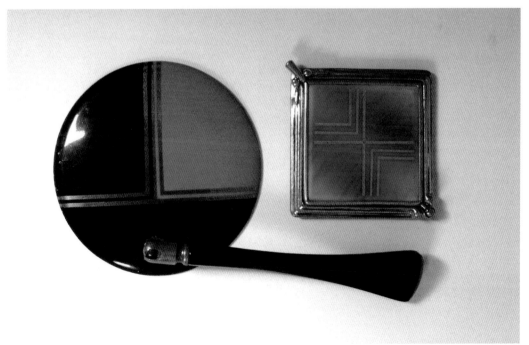

Art deco compact and mirror 1930s.

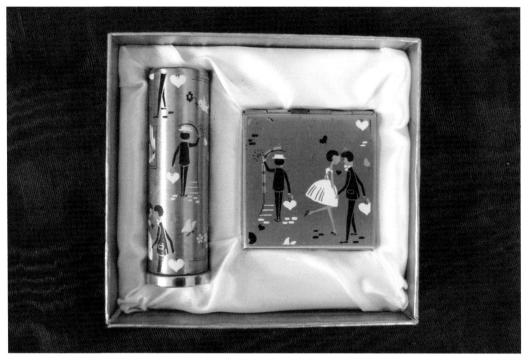

Mascot lipstick and pill box mint and boxed, 1960s.

Powder Compacts

Compacts are a well-established collectable. There are collectors' clubs both in the US and the UK and specialist reference books (see bibliography). As with all antiques, values depend on age, medium, design, maker and above all rarity. Unusual novelty designs and compacts in precious metals by big name jewellers typically command the highest prices: Salvador Dali's famous Bird-in-Hand compact recently fetched £1,800 at auction; in 2004 Sotheby's sold a Van Cleef and Arpels minaudiere for just over £6,000. Only a very limited number of pieces however will be worth four figure sums. At the other end of the scale, simple vintage compacts can be picked up for £10 or less; much is available for under £100, and even the more unusual designs are often priced in the low hundreds.

Some enthusiasts collect compacts of every style, others might focus on works from a particular period or by a certain maker. Compacts in interesting shapes, or decorated with popular themes such as ballet or animals (especially dogs) are perennially in demand. Certain pieces – for example military or golfing compacts – will have a crossover appeal to collectors in other areas which can make them more desirable.

Some compacts are unmarked; others will be inscribed with the name of a manufacturer or cosmetics company. Patent numbers can be traced to identify design, date and maker and silver marks can reveal where and when an object was made, and by whom. A good magnifying glass or jeweller's loupe and a book of hallmarks are both useful purchases.

Condition is crucial to value. Before buying, compacts should be examined both outside and inside. Because they were carried in a handbag, cases often became damaged – chipped enamel or scratched surfaces can be difficult or prohibitively expensive to restore. Hinges are another vulnerable area and cracked mirrors are hard to replace since modern mirror glass tends to be thicker than vintage. One solution is to cannibalise any missing or broken parts from another compact of the same type and period; and collectors will sometimes buy substandard pieces, purely to use for spares.

The presence of the original box, sifter (the mesh sieve covering loose powder), puff and any other contemporaneous material all add value and interest to a piece and a compact in mint and complete condition will always be worth more than a similar, less perfect piece. Sometimes however a certain amount of wear is unavoidable and the sense that an object has been used and loved can be partly what gives it its character.

Restoring and cleaning compacts should always be undertaken with care. Avoid abrasive polishes and never immerse a compact in water. A soft cloth sprayed with a little silicone polish can be used to clean surfaces; and silver cleaner should be used on silver compacts.

Cosmetics can sometimes damage or discolour their containers and many dealers and collectors will remove all traces of make-up (a dry toothbrush is useful tool for getting rid of powder). For other enthusiasts (myself included) part of the pleasure of a compact is the smell of powder and the brilliance of rouge. Cosmetics are part of the compact's history and if they are still intact, I leave them in. It goes without saying that vintage make-up shouldn't be worn. I tried a sample of 1930s cream rouge on my hand, 'natural and permanent', promised the tin and the last at least was true. It took three days, and more hand washing than Lady Macbeth, before the bright red colour wore off my skin. Never put anything on your face!

Powder boxes and tins
Powder boxes and tins can be beautifully decorated, and are collected both in their own right and to accompany matching perfumes and compacts. Desirable pieces include good art deco designs and well-known vintage brands: Bourjois' Evening in Paris for example, is very popular in the USA. Partly fuelled by nostalgia, demand is also growing for more recent products such as Kiku and Aqua Manda, favourite fragrances from the 1970s. Tins should be checked for rust and cardboard containers for damage and discoloration. When a box turns up mint and sealed with its powder intact do not open or empty it.

Lipsticks
Vintage lipsticks are collected in the US and interest is beginning to grow in the UK. Because this is a comparatively recent collecting area, prices are still very affordable. Simple pieces can be picked up for £2-5; interesting lip views and novelties for £10-£50 and only the rarest designs or examples in precious metals will fetch over £100. As with compacts there are many styles to choose from. Everybody produced lipstick cases, from cosmetics firms to compact makers to costume jewellers, and manufacturers competed with different decorations and opening mechanisms. Novelty designs are popular today as are iconic brands such as vintage lipsticks by Schiaparelli and Dior. It's not just the older metal cases that are collectable, but modern plastics. Certain classic 1960s designs by Revlon and Yardley are very sought after in the US, and Avon cosmetics attract dedicated enthusiasts.

As with compacts value is affected by condition. Sometimes lipsticks will be impossible to open – the top having fused to the base. While stick-on jewels can easily be replaced; damaged enamel and cracked plastic are often impossible to repair. Lipstick handkerchiefs and books of lip blotters make an interesting addition to a collection. Elaborate caddies, holding several lipsticks, were a popular American dressing table accessory in the 1950s and 60s and are collected for display purposes today.

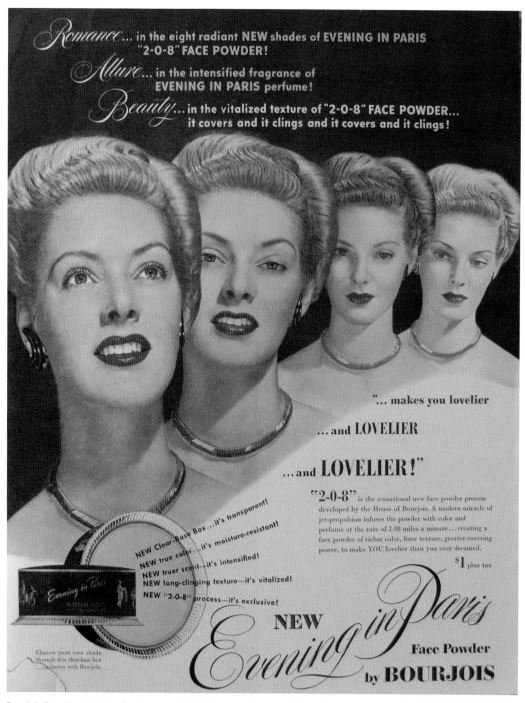

Bourjois Evening in Paris advertisement, 1947. Illustrates the powder box shown on page 239 and is a good example of how an advertisement can provide a useful tool for dates and information.

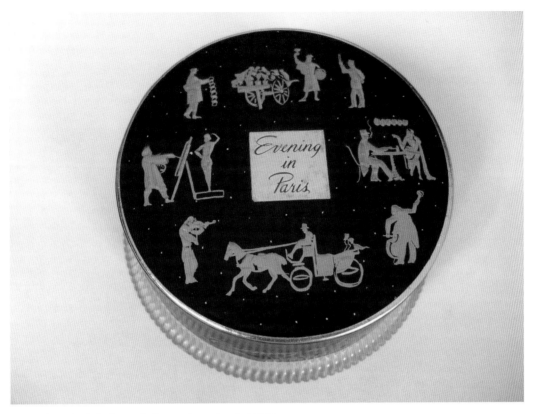

Bourjois' Evening in Paris powder box – mint and sealed, 1947.

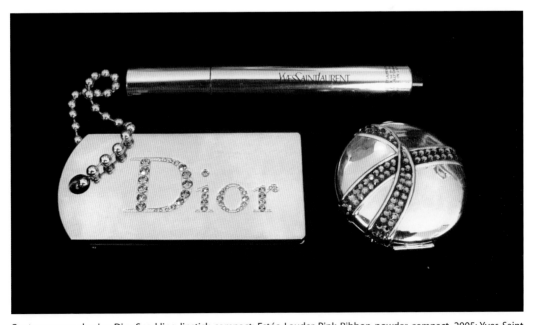

Contemporary classics: Dior Sparkling lipstick compact; Estée Lauder Pink Ribbon powder compact, 2005; Yves Saint Laurent Touche Eclat.

Ephemera

Ephemera provide a fascinating adjunct to a collection and can encompass anything from trade cards (promotional material printed by manufacturers to advertise their wares) to shop catalogues. For anybody interested in the history of fashion or beauty, vintage postcards of actresses and film stars illustrate who we wanted to look like and the latest trends in clothes, hair and make-up. These can be complemented by old photographs – snaps taken of and by ordinary people – less glamorous perhaps, but which demonstrate what most of us really did look like. Period magazines are very informative and an invaluable source for relevant advertisements.

Advertising and Packaging

Many cosmetic collectables, from bottles to tins to shop signs, fall under the category of advertising and packaging and can most easily be obtained from dealers specialising in these fields.

Vintage advertisements (taken from magazines and newspapers) are not only visually appealing but are a wonderful source of information, both about specific objects and the history of the day. Many vintage advertisement dealers trade online and for the collector, this has several advantages. Rather than leafing through endless magazines in the hope of finding a relevant ad., you can search directly by product name. Vendors also tend to catalogue their advertisements by subject, for example 'health and beauty' or 'vanity and grooming'. Whether you want to buy or not, for the cosmetic enthusiast this provides a library of pictures and information that would be very difficult to get elsewhere and that you can consult without leaving your computer.

Bottles and Pot Lids

From the second half of the Nineteenth Century, mass-produced white ceramic pots with transfer printed lids were used to contain everything from potted meat to toothpaste. Cold cream pot lids were manufactured in large numbers, and prices can range from £10–20 for commonplace designs to three figure sums for the most unusual pieces. Values are affected by design and rarity. Attractive images are popular; some chemist names are more desirable than others; and colour printed pieces (as opposed to the more usual black and white) also command a premium. Bear's grease containers are the most collected pot lids and can command high prices. Because of this, they have also been copied and collectors should beware of modern day reproductions.

Pot lids have often been rescued from Victorian rubbish dumps by bottle diggers and as with bottles, condition is all important to value. Huge numbers of bottles and jars were produced for the pharmacy. The name of skin washes and hair treatments was often impressed on the glass, but containers that still retain their original paper labels in good condition are sought after.

Modern Make-up – Saving the Empties

Many of us own a surprising, possibly embarrassing, number of cosmetics. A vintage collection can be supplemented with modern products. Get friends and family to pass on their discarded make-up and save any interesting packaging and ephemera. Obviously you can't keep everything (that way madness lies, and I should know). But it is worth holding on to good designer pieces, innovative or attractive novelties and perhaps a couple of objects that somehow encapsulate the makeup- mood of the moment. As we grow older, so the articles that we bought new become 'vintage'. Some of the compacts and cosmetics that we purchase today will undoubtedly become tomorrow's collectables. But what they will also provide is a snapshot of beauty practices at the beginning of a new millennium. A little bit of intimate and evocative 3D history – that you can see, touch and smell – and that will take women of the future back to their past and our present.

Bibliography

Allen & Ticknor (pub) – *The Toilette of Health* – Boston, 1934.

Angeloglou, Maggie – *A History of Make-up* – Studio Vista, 1970

Ayer, Harriet Hubbard – *A Complete and Authentic Treatise on the Law of Health and Beauty* (1899). *Woman's Guide to Health and Beauty* (1904).

Asser, Joyce – *Historic Hairdressing* – Sir Isaac Pitman and Sons ltd, 1966

Basten, Fred E. – *Max Factor's Hollywood:Glamour. Movies. Make-up* – General Publishing Group, 1995

Battiscombe, G. – *Queen Alexandra* – Sphere Books, 1972

Blakeman, Alan – *Miller's Bottles & Pot Lids, A Collector's Guide* – Miller's, 2002

Beerbohm, Max – *A Defence of Cosmetics. The Yellow Book, Vol. I.,* April 1894, pp. 65-82.

Braithwaite, Brian and Barrell, Joan – *The Business of Women's Magazines* – Asociated Business Press, 1979

Brett, David – *The Mistinguett Legend* – Robson books, 1990

Corson, Richard – *Fashions in Make-up* – Peter Owen, 2003

Cunnington, C.Willett and Phillis – *Handbook of English Costume in the 19th century* – Faber & Faber, 1970

Day, Ivan – *Perfumery With Herbs* – Darton, Longman & Todd, 1979.

De Castelbajac, Kate – *The Face of the Century* – Rizzoli, 1995

Druitt, Sylvia – *Antique Personal Possessions* – Blandford Press, 1980

Elms, Robert – *The Way We Wore* – Picador, 2005

Ewing, Elizabeth – *History of 20th Century Fashion* – Batsford, 1974

Etherington-Smith and Pilcher, Jeremy – *The It Girls* – Hamish Hamilton, 1986

Gerson, Roselyn – *Vintage Ladies' Compacts* – Collector Books, 1996

Gerson, Roselyn – *Vintage & Contemporary Purse Accessories* – Collector Books, 1997

Gold, Arthur and Robert, Fixzdale – *The Divine Sarah* – Harper Collins, 1991

Greer, Germaine – *The Female Eunuch* – Paladin, 1971

Gunn, Fenja – *The Artificial Face* – David & Charles, 1973

Haweis, Mary Eliza – *The Art of Beauty* – Harper, 1878

Houlbrook, Matt – 'The Man with the Powderpuff' in interwar London – the Historical Journal – Cambridge University Press, 2007

Howell, Georgina (ed.) – *In Vogue* – Conde Nast, 1975

Hulanicki, Barbara – *From A to Biba – The autobiography of Barbara Hulanicki* – V&A Publications, 2007

Keenan, Brigid – *The Women we wanted to look like* – Macmillan, 1977

Magnus, Philip – *King Edward VII* – Penguin, 1975

Marr, Andrew – *A History of Modern Britain* – Macmillan, 2007

Marsh, Madeleine – *Collecting the 1950s* – Miller's, 2004

Marsh, Madeleine – *Collecting the 1960s* – Miller's, 2004

Marsh, Madeleine – *Perfume Bottles – A Collector's Guide* – Miller's, 1999

Masden, Axel – *Coco Chanel* – Bloomsbury, 1990
Montez, Lola – *The Arts of Beauty, or, Secrets of a lady's Toilet. With Hints to Gentlemen on the Art of Fascinating* – J. Lovell, 1858
Mueller, Laura – *Collector's Encyclopaedia of Compacts, Caryalls and Face Powder Boxes* – Collector Books, 1997
Ovid – *Ars Amatoria* – translated by J. Lewis-May, Kessinger Publishing, 2005
Parkins, Wendy - *Fashioning the Body Politic* - Berg Publishers, 2002
Pharmaceutical Association – vol. 24 , March 1935
Pointer, Sally – *The Artifice of Beauty* – The History Press Ltd, 2005
Polhemus, Ted and Lynn, Procter – *Pop Styles* - Vermilion, 1984
Quant, Mary – *Quant by Quant* – Pan, 1966
Rimmel, Eugene – *The book of Perfumes* – Kessinger Publishing Co., 2004
Riordan, Teresa – *Inventing Beauty* – Broadway Books, 2004
Roddick, Anita – *The Body Shop Book* – Macdonald, 1985
Schroeder, Alan – *Josephine Baker* – Chelsea House Publishers, 1991
Scott, Linda M. – *Fresh Lipstick* – Palgrave Macmillan, 2005
Shrimpton, Jean – *An Autobiography* – Ebury Press, 1988
Staffe, Baroness – *The Lady's Dressing Room 1892* - Old House Books, 2006
Tapert, Annette – *The Power of Glamour* – Aurum Press, 1998
Tobias, Andrew – *Fire and Ice – The Story of Charles Revson – the Man Who Built the Revlon Empire* – William Morrow and Company Inc. New York, 1976
Turner, Alwyn – *The Biba Experience* – Antique Collector's Club, 2004
Twiggy by Twiggy – Granada Publishing, 1976
Watkins, Julian Lewis – *The 100 Greatest Advertisements* – Dover publications, 1959
Wayne, Jane Ellen – *The Golden Girls of MGM* – Robson Books, 2002
Webster, Thomas and Mrs Parkes – *Encyclopaedia of Domestic Economy* – Harper & Bros, 1855
Wood, Ean – *The Josephine Baker Story* – Hamish Hamilton, 1986
Woodforde, John – *The Strange Story of False Hair* – Routledge & Keegan Paul, 1971
Woodhead, Lindy – *Elizabeth Arden and Helena Rubinstein* – Virago 2004
York, Peter and Jennings, Charles – *Peter York's Eighties* – BBC Books, 1995
York, Peter – *Style Wars* – Sidgwick & Jackson, 1980
Cooper, Suzanne Fagence – *The Victorian Woman* – V&A Publications, 2001

Magazines, Newspapers and Journals across the decades including:
Alexandra Magazine
The Englishwoman's Domestic Magazine
Nova
New York Times
Punch
Queen and Harpers and Queen
The Guardian
The Observer
Times
Vogue
Woman Magazine

Index